BDJ Clinician's Guides

This series enables clinicians at all stages of their careers to remain well informed and up to date on key topics across all fields of clinical dentistry. Each volume is superbly illustrated and provides concise, highly practical guidance and solutions. The authors are recognised experts in the subjects that they address. The *BDJ Clinician's Guides* are trusted companions, designed to meet the needs of a wide readership. Like the *British Dental Journal* itself, they offer support for undergraduates and newly qualified, while serving as refreshers for more experienced clinicians. In addition they are valued as excellent learning aids for postgraduate students.

The *BDJ Clinicians' Guides* are produced in collaboration with the British Dental Association, the UK's trade union and professional association for dentists.

More information about this series at http://www.springer.com/series/15753

Tara Renton
Editor

Optimal Pain Management for the Dental Team

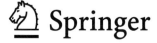 Springer

Editor
Tara Renton
Department of Oral Surgery
King's College London
London
UK

ISSN 2523-3327   ISSN 2523-3335   (electronic)
BDJ Clinician's Guides
ISBN 978-3-030-86636-5   ISBN 978-3-030-86634-1   (eBook)
https://doi.org/10.1007/978-3-030-86634-1

Cover illustration: Ella Renton

This Springer imprint is published by the registered company Springer Nature Switzerland AG
The registered company address is: Gewerbestrasse 11, 6330 Cham, Switzerland

Contents

1   **Introduction to Pain** 1
    Tara Renton

2   **Dental Pain: Dentine Sensitivity, Hypersensitivity
    and Cracked Tooth Syndrome** 9
    Nicholas Neil Longridge and Callum Cormack Youngson

3   **Chronic Pain and Overview and Differential
    Diagnoses of Non-odontogenic Orofacial Pain** 25
    Tara Renton

4   **Psychological Theories of Pain** 49
    Chris Penlington, Monika Urbanek, and Sarah Barker

5   **Psychological Interventions for Persistent Orofacial Pain** 61
    Sarah Barker, Monika Urbanek, and Chris Penlington

6   **An Overview of Dental Anxiety and the Non-pharmacological
    Management of Dental Anxiety** 69
    Jennifer Hare, Geanina Bruj-Milasan, and Tim Newton

7   **Medical Management of Dental Anxiety** 79
    Paul Coulthard

8   **Perioperative Surgical Pain Management** 89
    Nadine Khawaja

9   **Optimal Local Anaesthesia for Dentistry** 101
    Tara Renton

10 **Temporomandibular Disorders for the General
    Dental Practitioner** 123
    Emma Beecroft, Chris Penlington, Hannah Desai,
    and Justin Durham

11   An Update on Headaches for the Dental Team 141
     P. Chana and Tara Renton

12   Rhinosinusitis Update 153
     Claire Hopkins

Correction to: Optimal Pain Management for the Dental Team C1

Introduction to Pain

1

Tara Renton

Learning Objectives

- To understand the complexity of pain presentation in general and to be familiar with the benefits of a holistic approach in managing patients both with acute and chronic pain.
- To be familiar with advances made in understanding the pain mechanisms which are not to be overlooked.
- To gain some up to date tips on optimal acute pain management.
- To be familar with common orofacial pain conditions that can mimicking dental pain and lead to misdiagnosis.

The International Association for the Study of Pain (IASP) has defined pain as an unpleasant sensory and emotional experience associated with, or resembling that associated with, actual or potential tissue damage [1]. However, this does not reflect the functional, psychological and social implications of chronic pain. It proposes that pain can potentially occur with no physical damage or at the prospect of impending pain, i.e. a forthcoming visit to the dentist.

Your brain is the "boss" of pain, as without a brain you won't feel pain! Your little finger or big toe doesn't feel the pain, it's the brain's somatosensory cortex that overlays the pain experienced on the digit in danger, to effect appropriate protective behaviour, including removing your digit from harm. The brain informs whatever part of your body is getting hurt to move away from the cause. When this system is disconnected, that is when healthy healed tissue continues to "feel" pain, it is due to the brain continuing to overlay it upon the said digit. This in part explains how

---

The original version of the chapter has been revised. Spelling errors in Figure 1.1 were corrected. A correction to this chapter can be found at https://doi.org/10.1007/978-3-030-86634-1_13

T. Renton (✉)
Faculty of Dentistry, Oral & Craniofacial Sciences, King's College London, London, UK
e-mail: Tara.renton@kcl.ac.uk

T. Renton (ed.), *Optimal Pain Management for the Dental Team*, BDJ Clinician's
Guides, https://doi.org/10.1007/978-3-030-86634-1_1

chronic or pathological pain (also known as centralised or dysfunctional pain) arises in healthy tissues.

Although pain in response to tissue damage is a normal phenomenon, it may be associated with significant, unnecessary physical, psychological, and emotional distress [2, 3]. If a patient is phenotypically or genetically predisposed, pathological pain may result, with a continued overlay of pain in the digit or tooth by the brain. This may be neuropathic pain caused by nerve lesions (physical damage or lesional damage by systemic disease) or now called nociplastic pain related to multiple pain conditions such as TMD arthromyalgia, fibromyalgia, migraines, irritable bowel syndrome, interstitial cystitis, vulvodynia and other persistent pain conditions. The pain experience is dependent upon age, gender, ethnicity, culture, historic pain experience, personality, stress, depression and anxiety. Various settings can affect your pain levels including stress, anxiousness, tiredness and whether a patient has trust in the attending clinician. It is known that soldiers in military zones have higher pain thresholds in combat than off duty, and rugby players continue to score tries even after having just sustained a fracture during a tackle.

There have been significant developments in understanding the pain mechanisms and our response to them, the implications of which are spread over many different fields including neuroimaging, psychometrics, neuro-immunity, neurophysiology and pain genetics [4]. This in part may explain the difficulty in reaching and, or, maintaining a consensus for the taxonomy of pain itself. Woolf [4] eloquently highlights this by posing the question: "What is this thing we call pain?" Woolf classifies pain into three groups: nociceptive (detects noxious stimuli); inflammatory (adaptive and protective) which are now both combined into nociceptive pain; and pathological neuropathic with a lesion present or dysfunctional (now known as nociplastic pain) with no identifiable cause, shown in Fig. 1.1. In this paper it is emphasised that the processes driving these pain types are different and that treatments should be specific and preferably directed at the distinct mechanisms responsible [5]. Within the orofacial region there has been significant progress in advancing the understanding of musculoskeletal pain and neuropathic pain related to the orofacial region [6–10].

Orofacial pain (OFP) has been defined as pain whose origin is below the orbito-meatal line, above the neck and anterior to the ears, including pain within the mouth, and generally refers to non-odontogenic or acute pain [11]. The craniofacial region has a complexity of anatomic structures, and pain often radiates from one area to the other. As a result, the patient with orofacial pain may seek help from a number of specialists from different disciplines. Orofacial pain may present as a musculoskeletal disorder affecting muscles of mastication and cervical muscles, various neurovascular disorders such as headaches and vascular pains, and mimic various other conditions with aetiology from a host of other anatomic structures. The issues specific to trigeminal pain include the problematic impact on daily function. By nature of the geography of the pain (affecting the face, eyes, scalp, nose and mouth), it may interfere with just about every social function we take for granted. The trigeminal nerve is the largest sensory nerve in the body, representing over 50% of the sensory cortex. It is no wonder that pain within the trigeminal system in the face is often inescapable. However, due to a perceived low incidence of chronic orofacial pain

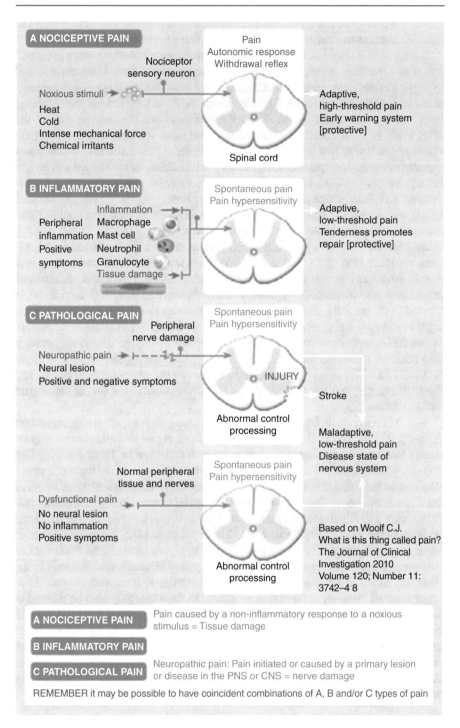

Fig. 1.1 Types of pain (Woolf et al. 2010)

conditions, many clinicians have a poor understanding of chronic pain, which can result in unnecessary surgery and occasionally harm to their patients.

Rather than a single nerve pathway, the term "trigeminal (three twins) system" refers to a complex arrangement of nerve transmission fibres, interneurons, and synaptic connections which process incoming information from the three divisions of the trigeminal nerve. The trigeminal nerve is a mixed nerve containing both sensory and motor fibres. Sensory fibres innervate the anterior part of the face, teeth, mucous membranes of the oral and nasal cavities, conjunctiva, dura mater of the brain, and intracranial and extracranial blood vessels. Motor fibres supply the muscles of mastication. Sensory information from the face and mouth (except proprioception) is carried by primary afferent neurons through the trigeminal ganglion, which is within the central nervous system (CNS), unlike other spinal sensory nerves where, the equivalent primary order ganglion bodies, lie in the distal root ganglia outwith the central nervous system (CNS). These primary order neurons then synapse with second-order neurons in the trigeminal brain stem complex (Fig. 1.2), which includes three separate nuclei proceeding in a rostral (superior) to caudal (inferior) direction: subnucleus oralis, subnucleus interpolaris and subnucleus caudalis. The subnucleus caudalis, the most caudal, is located in the medulla, at times extending to the level of C2 or C3 and is the principal brain relay site of nociceptive information arising from the orofacial region. While this complex receives afferent input primarily from the trigeminal nerve, it also receives afferent axons from the facial, glossopharyngeal, vagus and upper cervical (C2, C3) nerves. This connection between the upper cervical nerves and the trigeminal spinal tract nucleus may be a mechanism involved in facial pain and headaches [2].

Nerve fibres from different areas in the mouth may all synapse on another neuron (converge) in the spinal cord nuclei, thus sending a signal to the brain that may be poorly localised, explaining why early toothaches can often be difficult to pinpoint. Incoming pain signals to the subnucleus caudalis continue onto the thalamus where they can be modified (modulated) by descending nerve fibres from higher levels of the CNS or by drugs. The second-order nociceptive neurons in the subnucleus caudalis can be classified into two main groups: nociceptive specific (NS) neurons and wide dynamic range (WDR) neurons. These neurons have axons that form an ascending tract conducting nociceptive signals to higher levels of the brain for further processing. The next major synaptic connection in pain transmission is in the thalamus where axons traveling in the trigeminothalamic tract synapse with third-order neurons. Sensory information reaching the thalamus may also be relayed to several distinct nuclei in the thalamus. At the thalamic level, the action potential will be subjected to extensive processing through interactions among its various nuclei and by interconnections with the limbic, hypothalamic and cortical regions of the brain. It should be appreciated that until the nociceptive signal reaches the level of the thalamus, most of the reactions in the CNS have been reflex in nature. Only when the thalamus is involved, are the elements of consciousness and alertness introduced [2].

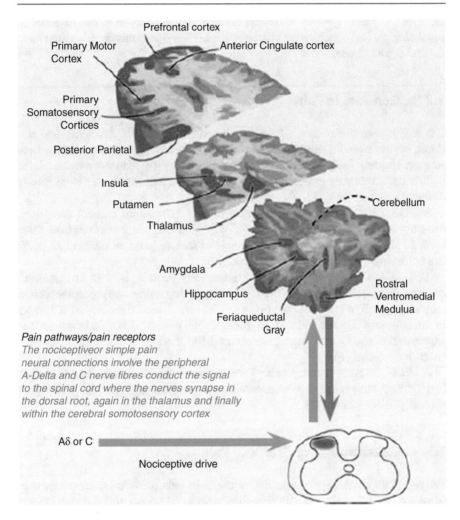

Fig. 1.2 Pain pathways in brain for general spinal sensory nerve

1.1   Pain Modulation

The human nervous system has an inherent ability to alter the intensity of nociceptive signals or reduce and increase the pain experience. This process is called modulation. There are several pain modulatory mechanisms: (1) endogenous opioid; (2) autonomic (serotonergic, dopaminergic, and noradrenergic); (3) inhibitory amino acid (cholecystokinin [CCK], galinin, and gamma aminobutyric acid [GABA]); (4) placebo; (5) nontraditional; (6) exogenous opioid; (7) cannabinoid and (8) electrical. The innate ability to downplay one's pain is likely to be due to genetics, psychological and conditioning characteristics. These mechanisms will be the basis for future pain management [6].

1.2   Genetics in Pain

It is well known that redheads have a melanocortin 1 receptor deficiency and as a result, are more predisposed to fear of pain and increased pain during injections and surgery. The deficiency of the Mu opioid receptor as seen in redheads may be related to 20% decreased pain thresholds. It does appear that redheads have a significantly different pain threshold [7].

SCN9A gene polymorphism resulting in Nav 1.7 sodium channel deficiency, resulting in total lack of pain perception, was identified in six children from three related Pakistani families. Although capable of feeling other sensations like warm and cold, they have a lack of pain perception.

The COMT (catechol-*o*-methyl transferase) protein is a brain "janitor" enzyme that metabolises the brain chemicals dopamine and norepinephrine. Dopamine is often known as the brain's "pleasure chemical", because of its role in transmitting signals related to pleasurable experiences. Variation in the expression of the COMT gene determines differences in pain directions experienced by patients [8].

A recent review of "neurogenetics" summarises some of the surprising aspects in highlighting the underlying susceptibility of certain individuals in developing chronic persistent pain [12].

1.3   Classification of Orofacial Pain

The recent international classification of orofacial pain provide 7 domains for orofacial pain [13]. The first domain is applied to acute "Healthy pain" is due to inflammation related to infection/autoimmune/trauma and stimuli (thermal/mechanical/chemical). Mechanisms and management of acute pain are covered in this series excluding local anaesthesia. The ICOP acute inflammatory pain domain is Orofacial pain attributed to disorders of dentoalveolar and anatomically related structures and includes:

- Intraoperative pain in the presence or absence of adjunctive sedation (for anxiolysis)
- Post-operative/post-surgical pain
- Pain as a symptom. The pain may be chronic (lasting under 3 months), usually a symptom of ongoing pathology.

ICOP include 5 further domains including; 2. Myofascial orofacial pain; 3. Temporomandibular joint (TMJ) pain; both of which can be acute or chronic in presentation. Where as domains 4-6 apply to more chronic conditions; 4. Orofacial pain attributed to lesion or disease of the cranial nerves; 5. Orofacial pains resembling presentations of primaryheadaches; 6. Idiopathic orofacial pain. Domain 7 is applied to the psychological consequences of the chronic pain in the orofacial region [13]. The Institute of Medicine (IOM) of the Health and Medicine Division of the National Academies of Sciences, Engineering and Medicine released a report and recommendations on chronic pain (www.nationalacademies.org/hmd on 6/29/2011). According to this report chronic pain affects at least 116 million American adults—more than the total affected by heart disease, cancer, and diabetes combined. Pain costs the nation up to $635 billion each year in medical treatment and lost productivity, making "the prevention of pain" the second major priority proposed for the nation's health improvement. An age-standardised analysis of 18 national surveys involving approximately 42,000 adults found that 37% of respondents in developed countries, and 41% in developing countries, reported a chronic pain condition [13].

Chronic orofacial pain syndromes represent a diagnostic challenge for any practitioner. Patients are frequently misdiagnosed or attribute their pain to a prior event such as a dental procedure, ear, nose and throat (ENT) problem or facial trauma. Psychiatric symptoms of depression and anxiety are prevalent in this population and compound the diagnostic conundrum. Treatment is less effective than in other pain syndromes, thus often requires a multidisciplinary approach to address the many facets of this pain syndrome [14].

Temporomandibular joint disorders (TMDs) are painful conditions of the temporomandibular joint (TMJ) and related structures excluding fractures and neoplasia. These represent both acute and chronic pain conditions.

Referred dental pain may be due to headaches, TMDs, angina, cervicogenic pain and oropharyngeal cancer.

1.4 Why Does Acute Pain Become Chronic Pain?

There are several hypotheses of how healthy acute inflammatory pain may "evolve" into unhealthy chronic pain. Persistent acute stimuli, for example, multiple surgeries or recurrent infections, causing central sensitisation, may increase the likelihood of developing chronic pain. Increased sensitivity of the CNS to peripheral stimulus is another demonstrated result caused by persistent inflammatory pain. Neuroplasticity relating to the interaction between the peripheral nervous system (PNS) and CNS results in permanent changes in the system and "memory of pain" caused by prior pain experiences, resulting in changes in the somatosensory cortex changes. Then of course there is increasing evidence for a genetic predisposition [15].

References

1. www.iasp-pain.org/.
2. Melzack R, Wall PD. Pain mechanisms: a new theory. Science. 1965;150:971–9.
3. Flor H, Elbert T, Knecht S, Wienbruch C, Pantev C, Birbaume N, Larbig W, Taub E. Phantom-limb pain as a perceptual correlate of cortical reorganization following arm amputation. Nature. 1995;375:482–4.
4. Woolf CJ. What is this thing called pain. J Clin Invest. 2010;120(11):3742–4.
5. Woolf CJ. Novel analgesic development: from target to patient or patient to target? Curr Opin Invest Drugs. 2008;9(7):694–5.
6. Kirkpatrick DR, et al. Therapeutic basis of clinical pain modulation. Clin Transl Sci. 2015;8(6):848–56.
7. Mogil JS. Pain genetics: past, present and future. Trends Genet. 2012;28(6):258–66.
8. Diatchenko L, Slade GD, Nackley AG, Bhalang K, Sigurdsson A, Belfer I, Goldman D, Xu K, Shabalina SA, Shagin D, Max MB, Makarov SS, Maixner W. Genetic basis for individual variations in pain perception and the development of a chronic pain condition. Hum Mol Genet. 2005;14(1):135–43.
9. Aneiros-Guerrero A, Lendinez AM, Palomares AR, Perez-Nevot B, Aguado L, Mayor-Olea A, Ruiz-Galdon M, Reyes-Engel A. Genetic polymorphisms in folate pathway enzymes, DRD4 and GSTM1 are related to temporomandibular disorder. BMC Med Genet. 2011;12:7.
10. Solovieva S, Leino-Arjas P, Saarela J, Luoma K, Raininko R, Riihimäki H. Possible association of interleukin 1 gene locus polymorphisms with low back pain. Pain. 2004;109(1–2):8–19.
11. Lopez BC, Hamlyn PJ, Zakrzewska JM. Systematic review of ablative neurosurgical techniques for the treatment of trigeminal neuralgia. Neurosurgery. 2004;54(4):973–82; discussion 982–3.
12. Cavalcante Felix FH, Fontenele JB. Neurogenetics can help turn pain concepts more objective. Pain Med. 2009;10(6):1147–8.
13. International Classification of Orofacial Pain, 1st edition (ICOP). Cephalalgia. 2020;40(2):129–221. https://doi.org/10.1177/0333102419893823.
14. Tsang A, Von Korff M, Lee S, Alonso J, Karam E, Angermeyer MC, Borges GL, Bromet EJ, Demytteneare K, de Girolamo G, de Graaf R, Gureje O, Lepine JP, Haro JM, Levinson D, Oakley Browne MA, Posada-Villa J, Seedat S, Watanabe M. Common chronic pain conditions in developed and developing countries: gender and age differences and comorbidity with depression-anxiety disorders. J Pain. 2008;13:883–91. https://doi.org/10.1016/j.jpain.2008.05.00.
15. Pureti MB, Demarin V. Neuroplasticity mechanisms in the pathophysiology of chronic pain. Acta Clin Croat. 2012;51(3):425–9.

Dental Pain: Dentine Sensitivity, Hypersensitivity and Cracked Tooth Syndrome

2

Nicholas Neil Longridge and Callum Cormack Youngson

Learning Objectives

- Explain the contribution of tubular fluid flow to dentinal sensitivity.
- Differentiate dentinal sensitivity from cracked tooth syndrome.
- Diagnosis and management strategy for the sensitive tooth.

It will be clear to all dental clinicians that dentine hypersensitivity is a very real issue affecting their patients, with one extensive study noting that the prevalence can be as high as 42% in young European adults [1]. It is also apparent that the sensitivity of any exposed dentine can vary considerably from patient to patient or even tooth by tooth within the same patient. The aim of this article is to explain why this may be the case, define hypersensitive dentine and consider a differential diagnosis for this condition, which should include a consideration of a cracked tooth. The article will also suggest strategies for dealing with hypersensitive dentine/teeth based on the underlying physiology of the tooth.

Even after many decades of investigation, there is still some debate as to the precise mechanism underlying dentinal sensitivity. A minority of authors consider that the extension of the odontoblast process throughout the dental tubule, coupled with "tight" and "gap" cellular connections between the odontoblast cell bodies, provides a mechanism for dentinal sensation. However, the hydrodynamic theory [2–4] has considerably the greatest support amongst the dental community and the likelihood of this theory being correct tends to be confirmed by the success of most topically applied desensitising agents [5].

N. N. Longridge · C. C. Youngson (✉)
University of Liverpool and The Liverpool University Hospitals NHS Foundation Trust, Liverpool, UK

Liverpool Health Partners, Liverpool, UK
e-mail: Nick.Longridge@liverpool.ac.uk; ccy@liverpool.ac.uk

Irrespective of the actual mechanism of dental sensation, it is often difficult to define objectively when dentinal sensitivity becomes "hypersensitive". In general terms, where the reaction to a normal stimulus is greater than expected, the subjective term "hypersensitive dentine" is used and there are a number of key reasons why this may be experienced. Hypersensitive dentine needs to be differentiated from the hypersensitive pulp caused by caries, so a thorough clinical and radiographic examination is required. However, in the absence of de novo or recurrent caries, the history of the condition and its nature will often clarify the diagnosis.

Before considering the diagnostic features further it is worth revisiting the structure and function of the dentine–pulp complex in health as these impact upon the perception of dentinal sensitivity.

2.1   The Structure of the Dentine–Pulp Complex in Health

The tissues that form the dental pulp and dentine are reliant upon migration of neural crest cells into contact with the oral epithelium [6] at around 10 days of gestation [7], with neural crest interactions also resulting in elements of the cornea and cochlea. The various interactions between the tissue layers responsible for tooth formation initially result in the differentiation of odontoblasts. This, ectomesenchymal derived tissue, then initiates ameloblast formation in the epithelial tissue leading to the formation of insensitive enamel. The ectomesenchyme in the dental papilla is therefore directly responsible for the development of both the dentine and the dental pulp. These sensitive tissues are thus, intrinsically, functionally and embryologically intimately related [8], even though their very different physical properties often make dentists think of them as distinct entities.

The dental pulp gains its sensitivity from the pulpal nerve supply and there are two main types of fibres responsible for pain sensation found in the pulp: myelinated Aδ, which tend to be concentrated more peripherally around the pulp chamber and unmyelinated C fibres. The latter, although distributed throughout the pulpal space, tend to be more concentrated in the central portions of the pulp [9].

Each cellular system within the pulp serves a purpose and it is becoming increasingly apparent that dental pulp mesenchymal cells, alongside fibroblasts within the pulp chamber, can differentiate into odontoblast-type cells to aid hard tissue repair and release a large number of factors affecting subsequent vascular and neural responses to inflammation.

The relationship of dental pulpal tissues to the dentine is represented diagrammatically in Fig. 2.1.

The dental pulp is a unique tissue enclosed, as it is, by dentine. As the root canal system, including the pulp chamber, is clearly unable to accommodate any substantial increase in the volume of the pulpal tissue, inflammatory responses of the pulp are restricted by the lack of ability for the tissues to swell. To compensate for this lack of compliance within the pulp chamber, arteriovenous shunts, which are particular to the dental pulp, can help to reduce the pulpal intracellular fluid pressure in the presence of inflammation [10].

Fig. 2.1 Dentino-pulpal
structure

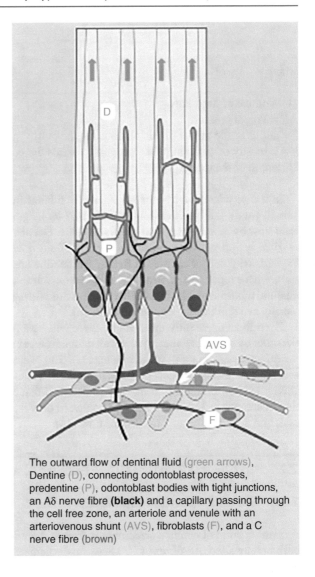

The outward flow of dentinal fluid (green arrows),
Dentine (D), connecting odontoblast processes,
predentine (P), odontoblast bodies with tight junctions,
an Aδ nerve fibre **(black)** and a capillary passing through
the cell free zone, an arteriole and venule with an
arteriovenous shunt (AVS), fibroblasts (F), and a C
nerve fibre (brown)

2.1.1   Dentinal Fluid Flows and Pulpal Sensitivity

There are several factors that are critical to the level of sensitivity of a tooth. In a
completely intact tooth (a closed system) there will be minimal outward fluid flow
from the dentine. However, when eating very hot or cold foods and drinks, convec-
tion currents within the tubular fluid will cause some shearing of the Aδ nerve fibres
adjacent to the tubule pulpal orifices, thereby providing some discomfort. This is
generally regarded as normal sensitivity of teeth.

Any factors which increase the rate of fluid flow will tend to result in greater
sensitivity and several of these are explained by the Poiseuille equation [11].

$$Q = \frac{\Delta P \pi r^4}{8 \eta l}$$

where

Q = volume of fluid flow
ΔP = Pulpal pressure
r = radius of the tubule (increases towards the pulp)
η = viscosity of dentinal fluid (increases towards the pulp)
l = length of the tubule

In a case where we assume no change in tubular fluid viscosity or pulpal pressure, a cavity that shortened a tubule to half its length would tend to increase the fluid flow by 32× compared to an intact tubule. Deepening that to one-quarter of its original length would result in an increased fluid flow by a factor of 1024×. This explains why deeper cavities in freshly cut dentine are much more sensitive (however, where reparative dentine has reduced or obliterated the pulpal aspect of the dentinal tubules, thereby markedly reducing fluid flow, carious dentine removal will usually be significantly less uncomfortable).

Even in an apparently intact tooth, there will be a fluid flow through dentine in the order of 18.1 pLs^{-1} mm^{-2} [12] as all dental tissues are slightly permeable (hence the effectiveness of tooth whitening agents). The overall tooth permeability can be increased by enamel defects (such as hypoplastic enamel) leading to increased sensitivity [13] of these teeth. It has been calculated that the threshold for pain sensation in humans is 3.92 nLs^{-1} mm^{-2} for outward flow (some 215× the "normal" flow rate) and 5.75 nLs^{-1} mm^{-2} for inward flow [14].

2.2 In Clinical Practice Other Factors Also Come into Play

2.2.1 Aδ and C Dental Pulp Fibres

A simplification of dentinal sensitivity is that fluid outflow stimulates the generally, peripherally sited, Aδ fibres [15]. These small diameter (1–6 μm), but myelinated, nerve fibres conduct action potentials relatively rapidly and so the perception of the pain related to short-acting dentinal fluid movement has a rapid onset, but also tends to resolve quickly.

In a more inflamed pulp, the C fibres (0.1–2 μm) also start to become more involved [15]. These are smaller unmyelinated nerves that conduct more slowly, but are stimulated by mediators of inflammation. These, initially, will tend to produce a less intense pain but one of longer duration.

In the absence of apical inflammation, without proprioceptive fibres being present within the pulp, the tooth concerned will be difficult for the patient to identify. At this point there will be stimulation of both Aδ and C fibres giving initial dentinal sensitivity, but with an associated longer dull ache.

When the pulp becomes more, and irreversibly, inflamed the concentration of mediators of inflammation will lead to apparently spontaneous episodes of dull throbbing pain often aggravated by local changes in blood pressure. The role of the Aδ fibres tends to become less prominent as the pulp becomes progressively inflamed, with temperature reaction becoming more mediated by C fibres [16]. Extreme sensitivity to heat may eventually develop as an end stage of reversible pulpitis, but with time this disappears, as the coronal pulpal tissue becomes progressively necrotic. More apically placed C fibres will now be responsible increasingly for pain conduction and, as inflammatory mediators diffuse from the pulp system into the apical tissues, the tooth becomes tender to apical pressure and the pain localisable due to stimulation of the many proprioceptive fibres that are present in the periodontium. Recent research continues to increase our understanding of the correlation between a clinical diagnosis of pulpitis and the histological status of the pulp. The identification that viable radicular pulp may often be present in cases of severe reversible and irreversible pulpitis has driven an interest in more conservative and biologically considered treatment modalities [17–20].

Paradoxically, the tooth may now appear non-vital, but it has been observed that C fibres (which do not respond readily to EPT [21]) can persist in tissues with low oxygen concentrations and conduct pain until complete pulpal necrosis occurs [22]. This explains the commonly encountered situation where, to all intents and purposes, a tooth considered to be non-vital is exquisitely tender to root canal instrumentation. In these circumstances, it is more accurate to describe the pulp as non-viable rather than non-vital.

2.2.2 Pulpal Fluid Pressure

This is important in the hydrodynamic theory of dentine sensitivity as the rate of fluid flow is linked to dentinal pain, and fluid under higher pressure will tend to move more rapidly outwards under the stimulus. Conversely, if an inward direction of fluid flow is initiated the pulpal pressure will rise further.

With an understanding of the neural, vascular and cellular responses to inflammation and the effect of pulpal blood pressure, a number of factors explaining dentinal sensitivity have direct clinical relevance.

Although most blood pressure effects occur in the circulation outside the pulp [10], the common finding that a toothache is worse when lying down, and often pulsatile, relates to the local increase of blood pressure in the tissues around the tooth, and slightly within the pulp. An increase in intrapulpal blood pressure will tend to increase fluid flows if (as is common) there are open dentinal tubules. This could be beneficial in preventing bacteria or their products from travelling down the tubules to cause further irritation, but the downside is that inflamed pulps are more sensitive than uninflamed.

Normal pulpal arteriole pressures are in the order of 40–45 mmHg [23], with lower pressures of 30–36 mmHg found in pulpal capillaries [4] and overall pulpal interstitial fluid pressures have been calculated as 14.1 cmH_2O (10.4 mmHg) [24].

However, in an inflamed pulp, the pressure may be as much as three times higher [25].

In the case of a normally intact but pulpally inflamed tooth (which therefore has a resultant increase in ΔP in the Poiseuille equation) being exposed to cold, there will be a marked outward movement of dentinal fluid and this will be experienced as pain [14] via Aδ fibre stimulation. In more irreversibly pulpitic teeth, however, it is often noted that cold can relieve discomfort. This may be explained by a transient reduction in the overall pulpal pressure due to dentinal fluid outward flow. Conversely, irreversible pulpitis is often aggravated by the application of heat. This is due to the net inflow of dentinal fluid into a pulp with an already elevated intrapulpal pressure, leading to increased C fibre discharge.

2.2.3   Alterations to Dentine

Dentine is a densely tubular structure with the number of tubules varying between facial, lingual and radicular surfaces but consistently higher more coronally [26]. For this reason, coupled with its proximity to hot and cold substances, most hypersensitive dentine is found around the cervical aspect of the tooth, where there has been the gingival recession and/or tooth wear but the more coronal enamel is intact.

Dentinal tubules are initially covered by; enamel, gingivae and/or cementum. However, trauma and gingival conditions leading to recession will expose large numbers [27, 28]. Factors that affect the fluid flow will include site of the tooth where tubules are exposed [26], the presence or absence of a smear layer [29] and the functional versus anatomic diameter of the tubules [30].

Hypersensitive dentine can be limited to a group of teeth, one tooth or even one aspect of a tooth, and is related to the fluid flow that is affected by the local dentine structure. Common aggravating factors are those which expose dentinal tubules that would otherwise be covered, e.g. gingival recession, erosion (from dietary or gastric acids) or abrasion.

The effects of these may also be modified by other factors that may have caused pulpal irritation including tooth whitening agents [31, 32] or trauma from the occlusion [33] as well as the response being affected by the environment (as both air and water are colder in winter).

It is worth noting that whilst attrition may also lead to the exposure of dentine, one response of this, usually a gradual process (which can also occur in slowly progressing dentinal caries) is the possible release of soluble growth factors that had been incorporated into the dentine matrix during its formation [34]. The subsequent diffusion of these (e.g. TGF-1, IGF-1, OP-1) down the tubules may stimulate the production of reparative dentine at the pulpal surface. Slowly progressive attrition is therefore seldom a cause of dentinal sensitivity. However, if this is coupled with erosion the rapid loss of tooth substance, greater than can be addressed by reparative processes, can have significant effects on sensitivity.

2.3   Erosion

The role of erosion in contributing to dentinal sensitivity has been recognised for many years [29], and a causal relationship has been demonstrated by the examination of a large dataset of patients with severe erosive toothwear [35].

Acid erosion of a dentinal smear layer, or other obstruction of the opening of a dentinal tubule is not always instantaneous, often leading patients to miss a cause-and-effect relationship. Whilst many drinks and foodstuffs (Table 2.1) are, by their nature acidic, few patients will suffer from immediate sensitivity as a result of direct contact (the general exception being where a cold acidic drink is swilled around the teeth rather than swallowed directly). Some alcoholic drinks are also acidic (Table 2.1) although, except in professional wine-tasters, the consequences are usually indirect.

Alcohol functions as a gastric irritant and, where the patient undergoes nocturnal or silent reflux, dentinal sensitivity will often take place the day following alcohol, rather than directly at the time of consumption. This is also often the case where the patient tends to eat a large meal just before sleeping (e.g. due to shift-working). A patient suffering from dentine hypersensitivity should therefore be questioned regarding the timing and size of their last meal of the day, to determine whether they are likely to suffer regurgitation during the night. As well as the timing and quantity it is worth asking what type of food is eaten—spicy foods also act as a gastric irritant leading to increased gastric acid secretion and an increased risk of reflux. A history of frequent antacid or proton-pump inhibitor use (e.g. Omeprazole) is therefore helpful to identify those at greater risk of dentine hypersensitivity.

Predictably, citrus drinks are particularly likely to aggravate the situation, due to the chelation of the citric acid to the hydroxyapatite. This can be aggravated by subsequent abrasion from toothbrushing where the toothpaste will be rendered more abrasive to the softened tooth surface. This is common where a "healthy breakfast" consists of a fruit salad followed by toothbrushing and so patients should be

Table 2.1 Common foodstuffs and associate acids

Foodstuff	Main acid constituent
Yoghurt	Lactic
Vinegars (including pickles and salad dressings)	Acetic
Ketchup	Acetic, phosphoric
Cola	Phosphoric, carbonic
Sports/energy drinks	Carbonic, citric
Wine—varies by grape variety	Tartaric, malic, pyruvic, α-ketoglutaric, fumaric, galacturonic
Cider	Malic
Coffee	Chlorogenic, citric, formic acetic, malic, glycolic, lactic, pyroglutamic
Fruit—varies by species	Citric, malic, quinic, tartaric, oxalic, α-ketoglutaric, lactic

encouraged to brush their teeth before breakfast or delay brushing for 30 min to allow some remineralisation from saliva.

As well as dietary (extrinsic) sources of acid, intrinsic sources of erosion from gastric acid are closely linked to voluntary or involuntary disorders e.g. gastro-oesophageal reflux disorder (GORD), bulimia nervosa, hyperemesis gravidarum. Patients with xerostomia (possibly secondary to medication) are also at increased risk due to the lack of remineralisation from saliva. Any patient who presents with dentine hypersensitivity should therefore be risk assessed for the likely contributing factors. However, irrespective of the source of the acid, the dissolution of any protective dentinal smear layer will lead to increased numbers of exposed dentinal tubules with a greater functional radius [5] and the risk of greater fluid flows (due to an increase in the πr component of the Poiseuille equation).

2.4   Clinical Management of Dentine Hypersensitivity

The ideal situation is where the causative agent is recognised and can be reduced by simple methods such as dietary modification. With time the dentine will become less permeable due to normal repair mechanisms, and the tooth return to normal sensitivity. Often however it is necessary to try to reduce the dentinal permeability on a temporary or more permanent basis. Use of desensitising toothpaste that may contain strontium acetate, calcium sodium phosphosilicate (CSPS), stannous fluoride or arginine calcium carbonate to occlude the openings of the dentinal tubules, can be effective [36]. Use of toothpaste containing potassium nitrate is also effective, possibly by diffusing down the dentinal tubules and blocking intra-dental nerve conduction [37]. Although a shortcoming of the occlusion of the tubules by toothpaste is their vulnerability to subsequent dissolution by acids or saliva, as well as being worn away by further toothbrushing or other abrasives, agents that precipitate intratubular crystals should be more effective for longer [38].

Professionally applied fluoride varnishes may also enhance hydroxyapatite formation in the tubules. Alternatively, a variety of resins, based on dentine-bonding systems, have been developed for dentine hypersensitivity where those form a polymeric barrier that is more resistant to subsequent acid dissolution. In more severe cases, placement of adhesive restorations can be indicated and, in extremis, root canal treatment. However, this, alongside extraction should be considered as a treatment of last resort.

In the absence of caries, alongside the diagnosis of dentine hypersensitivity, we should also consider whether the tooth is cracked.

2.5   Cracked Tooth Syndrome

The large number of literature reviews surrounding this subject is testimony to its enduring relevance to modern clinical practice, and the difficulty in diagnosing the condition [39–43].

There are a number of reasons why teeth crack, with contributions from anatomical, "iatrogenic" and even culinary factors. Cracked vital teeth often pose a diagnostic dilemma for the clinician as they can present in a patient who may also suffer from dentinal hypersensitivity but, even in the straightforward case, the apparently contradictory nature of the presenting symptoms complicates the definitive diagnosis.

Humans, uniquely, eat intentionally heated and chilled foodstuffs, often alternating between these during a meal. The thermal expansion and contraction of dental enamel lead to microcracks in this, naturally occurring ceramic-based material [44]. When coupled with low-frequency loading generated by chewing, there can be propagation of these enamel cracks. However, these are not usually problematic unless there is an additional underlying issue.

Intra-coronal dental restorations can contribute by weakening the tooth structure [45] and older cavity designs, employing sharp internal line angles, aggravate this even further by stress concentration. If a cusp is an excursive, functional or parafunctional contact, this makes a cracked tooth more likely to be symptomatic (Fig. 2.2).

Fig. 2.2 Sharp internal line angles in a tooth cavity predisposing to cusp fracture (arrowed)

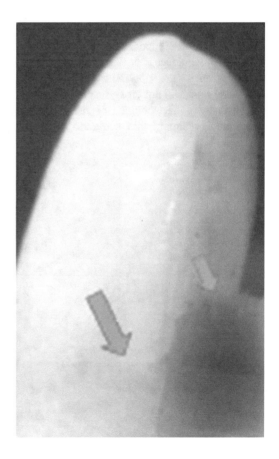

Whilst a careful examination of the functional occlusion is required, the diagnosis of a cracked tooth is often gained from the history, so a history of any trauma to the teeth or jaws should be elucidated at an early stage. Anatomically, upper first premolars are particularly prone to cracks running from the mesial to distal marginal ridges. This is partly due to their bicuspid occlusal form, but also due to the reduced coronaradicular bulk resulting from the presence of the mesial canine fossa, as well as a root furcation. Trauma from the opposing tooth (as a result of a blow to the lower jaw) or inadvertent biting on a hard material (e.g. as may occur with "granary" or stoneground bread) can therefore result in catastrophic fracture of this tooth (Fig. 2.3).

The pain history associated with a cracked tooth may appear confusing as it often contains elements that are strongly suggestive of dentine hypersensitivity but the patient will usually also complain of occasional tenderness on biting (but only with specific types of food), suggesting periapical periodontitis. However, the duration of the discomfort—which can remain severe and unchanged over many years—coupled with an absence of swelling or radiographic changes, can suggest nonodontogenic pain diagnoses such as trigeminal neuralgia or persistent orofacial pain. Radiographic examination usually fails to visualise the crack as it will tend to lie in the same plane as the film (mesiodistally). However, very occasionally, a buccolingual crack may be seen on a radiograph, usually in a lower molar (Fig. 2.4).

A far more predictable special investigation for a cracked tooth is transillumination, and a simple composite curing light can prove very effective in this regard. When using this technique, it is worth distinguishing small surface-level cracks (enamel crazing) from a more substantial crack involving dentine. In the latter case, the transilluminated light will not cross the crack line across the cusps. To further improve the effectiveness of this technique it is recommended that it should take place without the operating light shining into the mouth, to maximise the contrast (Fig. 2.5).

Fig. 2.3 Factors predisposing upper first premolar to fracture

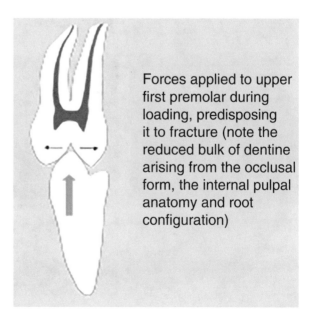

Forces applied to upper first premolar during loading, predisposing it to fracture (note the reduced bulk of dentine arising from the occlusal form, the internal pulpal anatomy and root configuration)

Fig. 2.4 Vertical crack (arrowed) visible on the radiograph of the lower right second molar

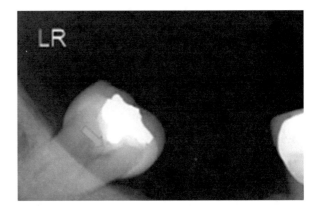

Fig. 2.5 Transilluminated lower right second molar demonstrating (incomplete) oblique fracture of mesial lingual cusp (Class II)

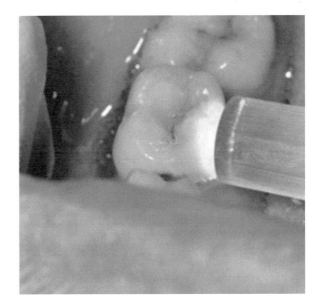

Once a crack has been identified, the next stage is to assess whether this tooth is responsible for the patient's pain. The patient can be asked to close firmly and slowly onto a resilient material (e.g. plastic saliva ejector or rubberised dental mirror handle) and then asked to open quickly. If the tooth is the one responsible, the identification is usually immediate. The mechanism behind this is illustrated in Fig. 2.6.

More refined tools, such as a FracFinder® or ToothSlooth® can help identify specific cusps contributing to the pain. It is worth bearing in mind that, where a blow has been received to the mandible, multiple teeth may have cracks and require treatment. However, the use of an orthodontic band can help to definitively assess whether a tooth is the cause of the patient's pain, by splinting the crack and allowing the patient to function unhindered between appointments thus confirming the diagnosis definitively (Fig. 2.7).

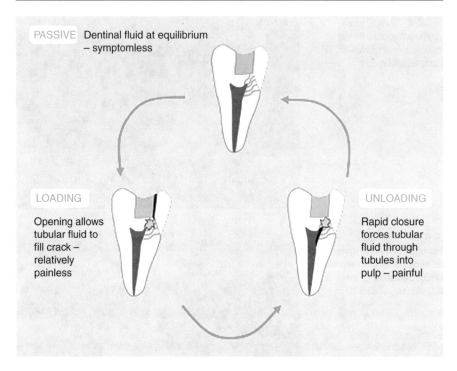

PASSIVE Dentinal fluid at equilibrium
         – symptomless

LOADING

Opening allows
tubular fluid to
fill crack –
relatively
painless

UNLOADING

Rapid closure
forces tubular
fluid through
tubules into
pulp – painful

Fig. 2.6 Mechanism explaining why pain is felt during 'unloading' when checking for a cracked tooth

Fig. 2.7 Temporary placement of orthodontic band to relieve symptoms and confirm diagnosis (same case as Fig. 2.5)

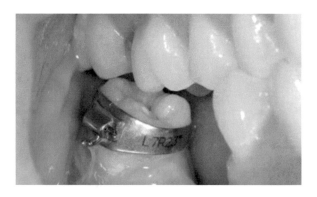

Having identified the tooth/teeth, a number of considerations have to be borne in mind to determine the prognosis. A simplified version of Talim and Gohil's classification of 1974 [46] can be applied to cracked tooth syndrome. Irrespective of whether the crack is incomplete, or complete, the prognosis tends to decline in the following sequence:

1. Crack is confined to enamel (class I)
2. Involving enamel and dentine but not involving the pulp (class II)

3. Fracture of enamel and dentine involving the pulp (class III)
4. A fracture involving the root (class IV)

When a crack terminates in a subgingival or subalveoar position rather than supragingival, it is more difficult to manage. Finally, the direction of travel (horizontal, oblique or vertical) can be superimposed upon this such that: a horizontal fracture of enamel only has an excellent prognosis; an oblique fracture of the enamel and dentine has a moderate prognosis; a fracture involving the pulp has a poor prognosis, but a vertical fracture involving the root has, effectively, a hopeless prognosis.

Unfortunately, there is still very little high-quality clinical research to be able to inform treatment decisions but, in general terms:

2.5.1 Single Cusp Fracture

1. Identifiable fracture extending supragingival (very good prognosis—remove cusp and restore [see Fig. 2.2]).
2. Crack extending obliquely subgingivally (moderate prognosis—reduce cusp height and overlay with adhesive restoration [47] to prevent further cusp flexure [see Fig. 2.5]).

2.5.2 Multiple Cusps

1. Mesiodistal or buccolingual where the supragingival extent can be visualised (good prognosis—remove fractured cusps and place an extra coronal* restoration [48]).

    It is recognised that extra coronal restorations are destructive of tooth tissue but the preparation shape tends to result in forces that "close" cracks during loading. Full crowns should be used where indicated but, following the principles of minimally invasive dentistry, alternative designs should be considered first. Simple occlusal coverage by resin-retained metal, in the form of a "bonnet" design, would be the least destructive design that would not produce opening forces on the crack. For aesthetic reasons ceramic may be preferred but will tend to be more destructive (due to the thickness required for the durability of the material). Whilst onlay restorations can be used in place of extra coronal restorations, it is best to use adhesive cavity designs that do not result in forces exerted during loading that would wedge the, already cracked tooth, apart.
2. Where the extent cannot be clearly seen, cut an occlusal cavity to determine the extent of the fracture. If it extends through the midline it is highly likely that root canal treatment will be required—especially if the crack continues into the roof of the pulp chamber. In these circumstances, the prognosis is moderate to poor. Root canal treatment and an extra coronal restoration will be required.
3. If, after commencing root canal treatment, the crack is seen to extend to the floor of the pulp chamber, the prognosis of the tooth is best considered hopeless.

References

1. West NX, Sanz M, Lussi A, Bartlett D, Bouchard P, Bourgeois D. Prevalence of dentine hypersensitivity and study of associated factors: a European population-based cross-sectional study. J Dent. 2013;41:841–51.
2. Gysi A. An attempt to explain the sensitiveness of dentine. Br J Dent Sci. 1900;XLIII:865–8.
3. Brännström M. Sensitivity of dentine. Oral Surg Oral Med Oral Pathol. 1966;21:517–26.
4. Orchardson R, Cadden SW. An update on the physiology of the dentine-pulp complex. Dent Update. 2001;28:200–9.
5. Seong J, Davies M, Macdonald E, Claydon N, West N. Randomized clinical trial to determine if changes in dentine tubule occlusion visualized by SEM of replica impressions correlate with in vivo assessment of tubule occlusion. Am J Dent. 2018;31:189–94.
6. Mitsiadis TA, Graf D. Cell fate determination during tooth development and regeneration. Birth Defect Res. 2009;7:199–211.
7. Nanci A. Development of the tooth and its supporting tissues. In: Nanci A, editor. Ten Cate's oral histology: development, structure, and function. 9th ed. Amsterdam: Elsevier; 2017.
8. Pashley DH. Dynamics of the pulpo-dentin complex. Crit Rev Oral Biol. 1996;7:104–33.
9. Fristad I, Bergreen E. Structure and functions of the dentin-pulp complex. In: Hargreaves KM, editor. Cohen's pathways of the pulp expert consult. 11th ed. Amsterdam: Elsevier; 2017.
10. Berggreen E, Bletsa A, Heyeras KJ. Circulation in normal and inflamed dental pulp. Endod Topics. 2010;17:2–11.
11. Pashley DH. Dentin: a dynamic substrate - a review. Scan Microsc. 1989;3:161–76.
12. Vongasavan N, Matthews B. Fluid flow through cat dentine in vivo. Arch Oral Biol. 1992;37:175–85.
13. Seow WK. Developmental defects of enamel and dentine: challenges for basic science research and clinical management. Aust Dent J. 2014;59:143–54.
14. Chaoenlarp P, Wanachantararak S, Vongsavan N, Matthews B. Pain and the rate of dentinal fluid flow produced by hydrostatic pressure stimulation of exposed dentine in man. Arch Oral Biol. 2007;52:625–31.
15. Yu CY, Abbott PV. Pulp microenvironment and mechanisms of pain arising from the dental pulp: from an endodontic perspective. Aust Endod J. 2018;44:82–98.
16. Närhi M, Yamamoto H, Ngassapa D, Hirvonen T. The neurophysiological basis and the role of inflammatory reactions in dentine hypersensitivity. Arch Oral Biol. 1994;39(Suppl):23S–30S.
17. Ricucci D, Loghin S, Siqueira J Jr. Correlation between clinical and histologic pulp diagnoses. J Endod. 2014;40:1932–9.
18. Hashem D, Mannocci F, Patel S, Manoharan A, Brown JE, Watson TF, et al. A clinical and radiographic assessment of the efficacy of calcium silicate indirect pulp capping: a randomized controlled clinical trial. J Dent Res. 2017;94:562–8.
19. Wolters WJ, Duncan HF, Tomson PL, Karim IE, McKenna G, Dorri M, et al. Minimally invasive endodontics: a new diagnostic system for assessing pulpitis and subsequent treatment needs. Int Endod J. 2017;50:825–9.
20. Duncan HF, Cooper PR, Smith AJ. Dissecting dentine - pulp injury and wound healing responses: consequences for regenerative endodontics. Int Endod J. 2019;52:261–6.
21. Närhi M, Virtanen A, Kuhta J, Huopaniemi T. Electrical stimulation of teeth with a pulp tester in the cat. Scand J Dent Res. 1979;87:52–8.
22. England MC, Pellis EG, Michanowicz AE. Histopathogic study of the effect of pulpal disease upon nerve fibres of the human dental pulp. Oral Surg Oral Med Oral Pathol Oral Radiol. 1974;38:783–90.
23. Matthews B, Andrews D, Wanachantararak S. Biology of the dental pulp with special reference to its vasculature and innervation. In: Addy M, Embery G, Edgar WM, Orchardson R, editors. Tooth wear and sensitivity. London: Martin Dunitz; 2000.
24. Ciucchi B, Bouillaguet S, Holz J, Pashley DH. Dentinal fluid dynamics in human teeth, in vivo. J Endod. 1995;21:191–4.

25. Heyeras KJ, Bergreen E. Interstitial fluid pressure in normal and inflamed pulp. Crit Rev Oral Biol Med. 1999;10:328–36.
26. Schellenberg U, Krey G, Boshardt D, Nair P. Numerical density of dentinal tubules at the pulpal wall of human permanent premolars and third molars. J Endod. 1992;18:104–9.
27. Gaberoglio R, Brännström M. Scanning electron microscopic investigation of human dentinal tubules. Arch Oral Biol. 1976;21:355–62.
28. Williams C, Wu Y, Bowers DF. ImageJ analysis of dentin tubule distribution in human teeth. Tissue Cell. 2015;47:343–8.
29. Pashley DH, Michelich V, Kehl T. Dentin permeability: effects of smear layer removal. J Prosthet Dent. 1981;46:531–7.
30. Michelich V, Pashley DH, Whitford GM. Dentin permeability: a comparison of functional versus anatomical tubular radii. J Dent Res. 1978;57:1019–24.
31. Anderson DG, Chiego DJ, Glickman GN, McCauley LK. A clinical assessment of 10% carbamide peroxide gel on human pulp tissue. J Endod. 1999;25:247–50.
32. Soares DG, Basso FG, Scheffel DS, Hebling J, De Souza Costa C. Responses of human dental pulp cells after application of a low concentration bleaching gel to enamel. Arch Oral Biol. 2015;60:1428–36.
33. Caviedes-Bucheli J, Azuero-Holguin MM, Correa-Ortiz JA, Aguilar-Mora MV, Pedroza-Florez JD, Ulate E, et al. Effect of experimentally induced occlusal trauma on substance P expression in human dental pulp and periodontal ligament. J Endod. 2011;37:627–30.
34. Kalyva M, Padadimitriou S, Tziafas D. Transdentinal stimulation of tertiary dentine formation and intratubular mineralization by growth factors. Int Endod J. 2010;43:382–92.
35. O'Toole S, Bartlett D. The relationship between dentine hypersensitivity, dietary acid and erosive tooth wear. J Dent. 2017;67:84–7.
36. West NX, Seong J, Davies M. Management of dentine hypersensitivity: efficacy of professionally and self-administered agents. J Clin Periodontol. 2015;42(Suppl):S256–302.
37. Markowitz K, Bilotto G, Kim S. Decreasing intradental nerve activity in the cat with potassium and divalent cations. Arch Oral Biol. 1991;36:1–7.
38. Arnold WH, Prange M, Naumova EA. Effectiveness of various toothpastes on dentine tubule occlusion. J Dent. 2015;43:440–9.
39. Gibbs JW. Cuspal fracture odontolgia. Dent Digest. 1954;60:158–60.
40. Guertsen W. The cracked-tooth syndrome: clinical features and case reports. Int J Periodontol Rest Dent. 1992;12:395–405.
41. Fox K, Youngson C. Diagnosis and treatment of the cracked tooth. Prim Dent Care. 1997;4:109–13.
42. Lynch CD, McConnell RJ. The cracked tooth syndrome. J Can Dent Assoc. 2002;68:470–5.
43. Lubisich EB, Hilton TJ, Ferracane J. Cracked teeth: a review of the literature. J Esthet Restor Dent. 2010;22:1–13.
44. Lloyd BA, McGinley MB, Brown WS. Thermal stress in teeth. J Dent Res. 1978;57:571–82.
45. Reeh ES, Messer HH, Douglas WH. Reduction in tooth stiffness as a result of endodontic and restorative procedures. J Endod. 1989;15:512–6.
46. Talim ST, Gohil KS. Management of coronal fractures of permanent posterior teeth. J Prosthet Dent. 1974;31:172–83.
47. Opdam NJ, Roeterrs JJ, Loomans BA, Bronkhorst EM. Seven-year clinical evaluation of painful cracked teeth restored with a direct composite resin restoration. J Endod. 2008;34:808–11.
48. Krell SKV, Rivera EM. A six-year evaluation of cracked teeth diagnosed with reversible pulpitis: treatment and prognosis. J Endod. 2007;33:1405–27.

Chronic Pain and Overview and Differential Diagnoses of Non-odontogenic Orofacial Pain

3

Tara Renton

Learning Objectives

- To familiarise dental practitioners with the latest knowledge on pain classification and diagnostic features.
- To equip dental practitioners with strategies to identify neuropathic versus inflammatory pain to prevent ill-advised surgery.
- To help to differentiate non-dental from dental pain.

Poorly diagnosed or managed pain in dentistry is the leading reported adverse event by dentists and by patients [1, 2] and the most common issue leading to complaints and litigation in the United States [1–4]. Although orofacial pain conditions mimicking dental pain are rare, the consequences are often severe for both the patient and the clinician [5]. Chronic orofacial pain provides a significant burden and remains poorly diagnosed and managed due to siloed training [6, 7], complex anatomy and the plethora of conditions that can present above the neck. The dentist's role in diagnosing and managing the patient's pain involves several aspects of patient care:

- Diagnosing and managing routine dental and surgical pain correctly.
- Identifying cancer-induced pain or referred pain [8] and referring appropriately (up to 20% of patients experience pain prior to diagnosis of oropharyngeal cancer) [7].
- Recognising non-odontogenic pain and preventing inappropriate dental care.
- Preventing nerve injuries related to dental treatment resulting in chronic post-surgical pain.

The original version of the chapter has been revised. Spelling error in Figure 3.1 was corrected. A correction to this chapter can be found at https://doi.org/10.1007/978-3-030-86634-1_13

This article may contain repetition when read in conjunction with other articles in this issue as they are designed to be read independently.

T. Renton (✉)
Faculty of Dentistry, Oral and Craniofacial Sciences, King's College London, London, UK
e-mail: Tara.renton@kcl.ac.uk

© The Author(s), under exclusive license to Springer Nature Switzerland AG 2022, corrected publication 2023
T. Renton (ed.), *Optimal Pain Management for the Dental Team*, BDJ Clinician's Guides, https://doi.org/10.1007/978-3-030-86634-1_3

The third role in pain management is particularly challenging as dentists have limited knowledge of common headaches and sinus conditions. There are several types of pain: healthy nociceptive and inflammatory pains that are the "bread and butter" of dental care, and the unhealthy non-protective pains including neuropathic with or without autonomic components and dysfunctional or centralised pain (Fig. 3.1) [9]. In 1993, an estimated 12.2% of the American general population had experienced toothache in the last 6 months [10]. In the United States between 1997 and 2000, 2.95 million people presented to an emergency department with a chief complaint of toothache or dental injury [10].

The chronic pains reflect a disease of the peripheral and/or central system, whereby after the tissue injury has healed, the brain continues to overlay pain in the healthy region causing chronic pain perception in healthy tissues. There are several types of pain and two or three types of chronic pain, depending upon the mechanistic differentiation (Fig. 3.1). Chronic pain propensity may infer that a patient may have a phenotypic and or genotypic predisposition for developing chronic pain, many factors for which have been reported in relation to chronic postsurgical pain [11].

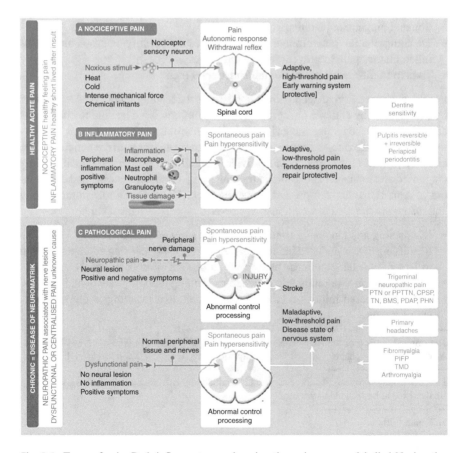

Fig. 3.1 Types of pain. Both inflammatory and nociceptive pain are now labelled Nociceptive pain. Neuropathic pain defined as a lesion of or damage to the somatsensory syste remains unchanged and dysfunctional pain is now termed Nocicplastic pain (Based on Woolf [9])

It has been recognised that genetic and psychological backgrounds are risk factors for patients being vulnerable to developing chronic pain states.

Toothache and dental pain can present in many guises (Fig. 3.2). Elicited pain seen in reversible pulpitis with touch and cold can mimic trigeminal neuralgia, post-traumatic neuropathies, trigeminal autonomic cephalalgias and other secondary neuropathies.

The dull episodic intense throbbing pain of irreversible pulpitis can mimic myofascial pain and migraine.

Dentists may be unfamiliar with chronic pain and as a result, may often overlook the possibility of non-odontogenic pain rather than healthy toothaches. After all, the toothache is the most common OFP and should be considered and subsequently dismissed in the first instance. Vitality tests are notoriously unpredictable, often not

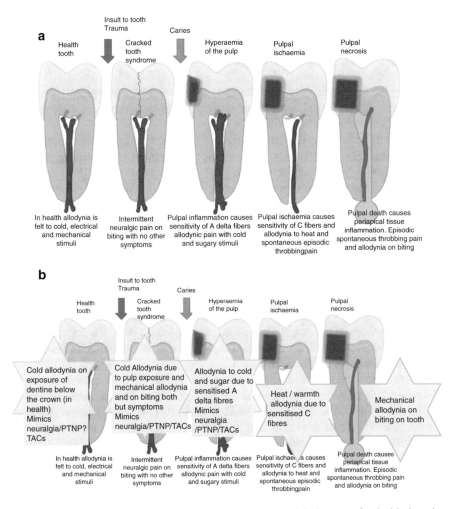

Fig. 3.2 Toothache presents in various forms due to various clinical stages of pulpal ischaemic and viability. You must consider that all presentations may be present is a multirooted molar posterior tooth (**a**) Toothache can mimic neuralgic conditions (**b**) and headache conditions (**c**)

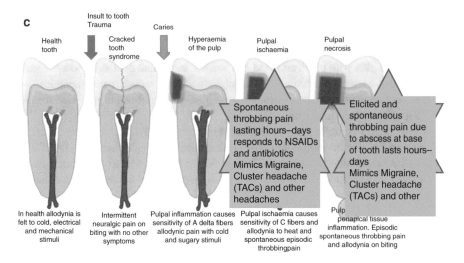

Fig 3.3 (continued)

resolving the diagnostic dilemma but adding to it, indicating non-vitality in an unrestored, non-diseased vital tooth often leading the desperate patient and clinic to make irrational treatment decisions.

What is also counterintuitive for dentists is that they are familiar with mechanical allodynia and hyperalgesia (pain to non-nociceptive stimuli and increased pain to a painful stimulus [normal in dentine sensitivity and pulpal sensitivity]) in health. No other human organ displays these conditions in health only with inflammation present. Thus, neuralgic oral pain can be present in health; dentine sensitivity or exposed pulp as well in many other pathological conditions (odontogenic infections, salivary obstructive disease, temporomandibular disorders (TMD) dysfunctional disc entrapment, mucosal ulceration, trigeminal autonomic cephalalgias (TACs), referred cancer pain, trigeminal neuralgia (TN) and post-traumatic neuropathy, making the diagnosis of OFP conditions challenging.

Another challenge for dentists in diagnosing non-odontogenic pain includes an ageing population with heavily restored restorations, vitality tests that are notoriously unpredictable and limited education about chronic pain, leading dentists to remain unfamiliar with chronic pain and as a result may often overlook the possibility of neuropathic or neurovascular pain.

There were contesting OFP classification provided by the International Headache Society (IHS) [12], International Craniofacial Disorders Classification (ICHD-3) [13], American Academy of Orofacial Pain (AAOP) [14], American Academy of Craniofacial Pain (AACP) [15] and the International Association for the Study of Pain (IASP) [16]. There is now the International Classification of Orofacial Pain (ICOP), which is endorsed by the stakeholders mentioned above [17]. There are seven domains; 1. Orofacial pain attributed to disorders of dentoalveolar and anatomically related structures; 2. Myofascial orofacial pain; 3. Temporomandibular joint (TMJ) pain; 4. Orofacial pain attributed to lesion or disease of the cranial nerves; 5. Orofacial pains resembling presentations of primary headaches; 6. Idiopathic orofacial pain and 7. Psychosocial assessment of patients with orofacial pain. These domains are a mixture

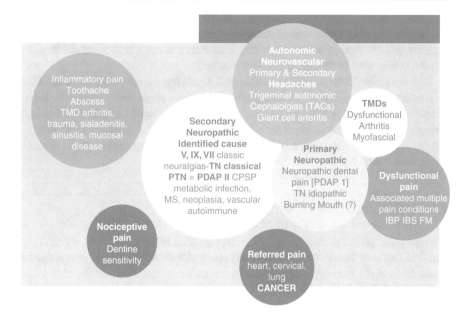

Fig. 3.3 Types of orofacial pain

of anatomical and mechanistic groupings [17]. The author suggests a simplified mechanistic classification (Fig. 3.3). This article will address these various types of non-odontogenic pain and how they may mimick toothache in the following order:

- Non-odontogenic inflammatory pain
- Referred or heterotropic pain (not included in ICOP)
- Temporomandibular disorder pain after TMDs (myalgia, arthralgia and myofascial)
- Neurovascular pain after neurvascular pain (primary headaches)
- Neuropathic pain (primary and secondary)
- Idiopathic pain

3.1   Inflammatory Pain

Acute Rhinosinusitis can be associated with causing toothache symptoms [18]. The sinus, allergy and migraine study (SAMS) highlighted the diagnostic difficulty as pain presented in 1.6% maxillary unilateral, 1.6% bilateral maxillary and the second division and third division of the trigeminal nerve (V2 and V3) unilateral in 3.2% of cases [19]. It is well recognised by dentists that sinusitis can mimick dental pain however, up to 88% of people who self-report or have physician-diagnosed sinusitis actually have a maxillary migraine [20, 21]. You can read more about Rinosinusitis in the dedicated chapter.

Sinusitis mimicking toothache: The episodic and or continuous fluctuant pain of sinusitis classically worsens on posturing forward and increased barometric pressure. The dull fluctuant ache can present as maxillary molar or premolar pain, which may also respond to anti-inflammatories and antibiotics. Panoramic radiographs are not reliable in diagnosing antral mucosal thickening in association with chronic sinusitis and, as mentioned above, a key differential diagnosis that should be considered is migraine in the maxillary distribution.

Salivary gland Sialadenitis may cause pain overlying the mandibular region. Due to the nature of obstructive salivary gland disease, it can present as episodic high-intensity pain and may respond to antibiotics. The additional features of mealtime syndrome, discharge from ducts salivary calculate present or discharge and tenderness of the glands may confirm that the pain is related to salivary gland disease rather than dental pain.

3.2   Referred (Heterotropic) Pain

Cervicogenic pain referred to the orofacial region: The potential for cervical dysfunction to cause headache is recognised under the classification of cervicogenic headache, and the pain typically manifests within the dermatomes of the trigeminal and upper cervical (C2, C3) nerves. C2–3 provides a general sensation over the skin at the angle of the mandible [22].

Cardiac heterotropic pain: "Toothache pain" of angina origin has been frequently reported [24], and can be bilateral [25], though mainly reported on the left side [26].

The cardiac innervations depend on the afferent sympathetic and parasympathetic (PS) nerves. Most of the innervations are transferred via the first five thoracic roots, causing pain in the chest and arms, but not in the face and jaw. For this reason, it is thought that the parasympathetic system has a significant role in causing mandibular pain, via the trigeminal nucleus [27, 28].

Angina-related facial pain is likely to present concomitantly with left arm and chest pain but can arise alone. The pain is likely associated with excursion and alleviated on rest or on using medication for angina. The patient will have risk factors associated with ischaemic heart disease and may or may not be diagnosed with angina [8]. The clinician should always exclude exercise induced left sided facial pain. Referral to the patient's medical practitioner is recommended if suspected.

Giant cell arteritis should be suspected in patients older than 50 years who present with persistent headaches centred on one or both temples. It is associated with cold temperatures, visual acuity changes during attacks and jaw claudication. The examination may reveal an enlarged, tender temporal artery. Laboratory investigation should include erythrocyte sedimentation rate and/or C-reactive protein.

Pain-related to giant cell arteritis is generally distributed in the first division of the trigeminal nerve (V1) distribution but can radiate to V2 and V3. The pain is intense and excruciating with or without visual signs. The temporal artery affected may be prominent and tender to palpation. Urgent referral of the patient is required for assessment and steroid medication to prevent blindness.

Oropharyngeal carcinoma: referred to pain presenting as toothache in the posterior mandible. Missing a cancer diagnosis is not only a serious event and also results in complaints and fitness to practise investigations for those dentists involved. We are taught that oral cancer presents painlessly, however, recent studies have

Table 3.1 Red flags for cancer

(NICE recommend immediate referral to a relevant specialist and maximum 2-week wait for consultation)
Systemic signs
• Over 50 years
• Previous history of carcinoma
• Smoking/alcohol/betel nut/paan
• Night fevers
• Weight loss
• Blood loss/anaemia
Local signs
• Recent onset
• Rapid growth
• Neuropathy—sensory or motor
• Resorption of adjacent structures
• Localised mobility of teeth
• Progressive trismus
• Persistent painless ulcer
• Lymphadenopathy—painless, persistent
• Lack of response to conventional treatments:
– Antibiotics
– Endodontic surgery

highlighted that pain often precedes the diagnosis of oral and oropharyngeal carcinoma. The pain was the initial symptom of oral cancer in 19.2% of 1412 patients including 12 different complaints including sore throat (37.6%), tongue pain (14.0%), mouth pain (12.9%); pain when swallowing (11.1%), dental pain (5.9%); earache (5.9%); pain in the palate (4.1%); burning mouth (3.3%); gingival pain (2.2%); pain when chewing (1.1%); neck pain (1.1%) and facial pain (0.7%) [29]. In another study, 12 patients experienced a recurrence of primary head and neck cancers preceded by severe OFP. The pain began within 6 months following treatment in 10 of 12 patients and was progressive in 11 of 12 patients [30].

With oropharyngeal cancer being one of three cancers increasing in prevalence (along with melanoma and hepatocellular cancer) and association with human papillomavirus (HPV) and oral sex [31], the dental profession must be aware of oropharyngeal cancer presenting as pain mimicking rare OFP conditions, for example glossopharyngeal neuralgia, preauricular pain and jaw pain.

If the patient presents with recent onset pain symptoms, particularly with risk factors, for example, sensory or motor neuropathy (Table 3.1 Red Flags for neoplasia), neoplasia must be first excluded before continuing dental treatment.

3.3 Temporomandibular Disorder Pain

TMDs can be subcategorised into three groups: arthrogenuous and myogenous and and headaches related to TMDs [31].

The most common chronic pain conditions presenting in the orofacial region are TMDs followed by headaches [32]. There is significant chronic pain comorbidity in patients with TMD [33]. Both of these conditions can refer pain to the second

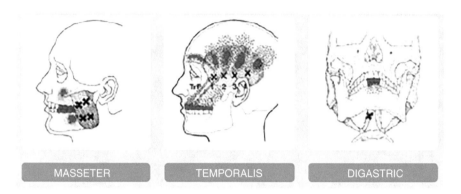

Fig. 3.4 Referral pain patterns from masticatory muscles [23]

and third division of the trigeminal nerve mimicking toothache, emphasising the importance for dental practitioners to understand the possibility of TMD myofascial pain mimicking posterior maxillary and mandibular molar pain [23, 32].

Myofascial pain related to TMDs can be referred to as maxillary and mandibular molar teeth (Fig. 3.4). Please see the dedicated chapter on TMDs by Justin Durham and team.

3.4   Neurovascular Pain

3.4.1   Primary Headaches (Table 3.2)

There are several reports of headaches resulting in dental pain mistakenly treated with dental restorations, root canal treatments and resultant extractions which, unsurprisingly, do not result in pain resolution. The International Classification of Orofacial Pain [17] now includes a domain dedicated to neruovascular, primary headaches presenting in the maillary and mandibular divisions of the trigeminal nerve. The dental team must be aware of particulalry migraine affecting teh maxilla and mandibular regions often mimicking dental interittent throbbing pain.

Migraines: Migraine headache sites are usually temporal, supraorbital, frontal, retrobulbar, parietal, auricular and occipital. However, they may occur in the malar region and upper and lower teeth base of nose and median in migraine is also reported [19, 34]. It is well recognised by dentists that sinusitis can mimic dental pain, however, up to 88% of people who self-report or have physician-diagnosed sinusitis actually have V2 migraine [20, 21].

Migraine diagnostic criteria are specific [12, 13], and associated signs include nausea, dizziness, photophobia phonophobia, tinnitus, visual aura and numbness. The pain is characteristically throbbing and mainly unilateral in V1 distribution but can present bilaterally. There is often a family history of migraines, and the prevalence in females is increased. Migraine headache sites are usually temporal, supraorbital, frontal, retrobulbar, parietal, auricular and occipital.

Table 3.2 Diagnostic criteria for primary headaches

Condition	Classification system	Diagnostic criteria ICHD https://www.ichd-3.org/how-to-use-the-classification/
Primary headaches		
Migraine	ICHD-3 Part 1 Section 1.1-2	**Description**: Migraine has two major subtypes. 1.1 Migraine without aura is a clinical syndrome characterized by headache with specific features and associated symptoms. 1.2 Migraine with aura is primarily characterized by the transient focal neurological symptoms that usually precede or sometimes accompany the headache. Some patients also experience a premonitory phase, occurring hours or days before the headache, and a headache resolution phase. Premonitory and resolution symptoms include hyperactivity, hypoactivity, depression, cravings for particular foods, repetitive yawning, fatigue and neck stiffness and/or pain.
Neurovascular pain or neuropathic with autonomic signs		
Trigeminal Autonomic Cephalalgia	ICHD-3 Part 1 Section 3.1-5	**Description**: The trigeminal-autonomic cephalalgias (TACs) share the clinical features of headache, which is usually lateralised, and often prominent cranial parasympathetic autonomic features, which are again lateralized and ipsilateral to the headache. Experimental and human functional imaging suggests that these syndromes activate a normal human trigeminal-parasympathetic reflex, with clinical signs of cranial sympathetic dysfunction being secondary. **Types** 3.1 Cluster headache 3.2 Paroxysmal hemicrania 3.3 Short-lasting unilateral neuralgiform headache attacks 3.4 Hemicrania continua 3.5 Paroxysmal hemicrania

Pain can be initiated by surgical intervention in most of the patients similar to a previous study including two patients with migraine precipitated or aggravated by dental treatment [35] reporting that one of two patients said: "it's like my old migraine's moved to my face". In addition, this study highlighted that both patients were scheduled for interventional pain management procedures which would likely have been detrimental. The peripheral afferent barrage from the second and third division of the trigeminal nerve onto second-order neurons in the trigeminal nucleus following an acute injury to the face or jaw may induce a central change in the processing of nociceptive signals from the head and neck that leads to a "remapping" of the pain associated with subsequent migraine events [35, 36]. This relocation or remapping of the migraine pain may also alter the expressed associated symptoms and further impede the diagnosis.

Migraine can mimick dental pain as V2 and V3 branches of the trigeminal nerve supply temporal meninges [37].

It is reported that migraine can commonly present in the second and third division of the trigeminal system [34, 38]. A study of 517 migraine patients in Germany reported that 46 (8.9%) cases of migraine pain involved the head and the lower half of the face. Patients with facial pain suffer more trigeminal-autonomic symptoms than migraine patients (47.8% vs. 7.9%; $P < 0.001$). In one case isolated facial pain without a headache was the leading symptom of migraine [34]. There are several reports of migraines resulting in dental pain mistakenly treated with dental restorations, root canal treatments and resultant extractions which, unsurprisingly do not result in pain resolution in two cases [36], and seven cases [39]. Due to the variable presentation of toothache (hyperaemic pulp causing initially elicited neuralgia with cold and mechanical allodynia, subsequent pulpal death resulting in sensitivity to heat and spontaneous throbbing aching pain) many chronic pain conditions can be mistakenly diagnosed, for example, trigeminal autonomic cephalalgia due to cracked tooth syndrome [39].

Unfortunately, due to the lack of taking down a simple pain history that includes migrainous associated signs or past history of headaches, these patients were exposed to continued dental and or ENT invasive procedures and inappropriate medication [40]. You can read more about primary headaches in the chapter on Primary Headaches.

Trigeminal autonomic cephalalgias (TACs) are conditions including cluster headaches.

Presentation: These neurovascular conditions present with severe intense multiple unilateral neuralgic stabbing pains (suicidal pain), mainly in the V2, peri retroocular region, with associated autonomic signs including ptosis, meiosis, conjunctival irritation, unilateral nasal congestion with cheek flushing on the side of pain. The prevalence in males is increased. The pain is episodic, unilateral, very high intensity, often multiple neuralgic stabs on a background of intense burning pain behind the eye. Unlike migraine, where patients curl up in a dark quiet room not wanting to move, patients experiencing TAC pain are severely agitated, related to hypothalamic behaviour [40].

Mimicking toothache: The regions of the orofacial region most commonly affected by neurovascular pain include the premaxilla (30%), V2 (17%), V3 (31%) with pain duration of 9–16 h occurring mainly in men [41].

Patients with TACs will often consult dentists (34–45%) and ENT consultants (27–33%), with an average of 4.3 physicians consulted prior to diagnosis with 4% of patients undergoing sinus surgery; 15% of paroxysmal hemicrania patients have pain similar to dental pain [40, 41].

Many patients previously diagnosed with persistent idiopathic facial pain were likely suffering from migraines and or TACs. Because of the episodic nature, there maybe a response to treatment: caution is advised. It is essential that practitioners enquire about associated migrainous and autonomic signs.

3.5   Neuropathic Pain (NP)

NP (Table 3.3) is the result of injury to nerve fibres due to various aetiologies including toxic, traumatic, ischaemic, metabolic, infectious or compressive damage [42]. Positive symptoms are typically altered or painful sensations such as tingling,

Table 3.3 Diagnostic criteria for neuropathic pain conditions

Condition	Classification system	Diagnostic criteria ICHD https://www.ichd-3.org/how-to-use-the-classification/
1 Neuropathic pain		
Painful Post Traumatic Neuropathy PPTN	ICOP Domain 4 Neuropathic	**Previously used terms:** Anaesthesia dolorosa; painful post-traumatic trigeminal neuropathy. Description: Unilateral or bilateral facial or oral pain following and caused by trauma to the trigeminal nerve(s), with other symptoms and/or clinical signs of trigeminal nerve dysfunction, and persisting or recurring for more than 3 months **Diagnostic criteria:** A. Pain, in a neuroanatomically plausible area within the distribution(s) of one or both trigeminal nerve(s), persisting or recurring for >3 months and fulfilling criteria C and D B. Both of the following: 1. History of a mechanical, thermal, radiation or chemical injury to the peripheral trigeminal nerve(s) 2. Diagnostic test confirmation of a lesion of the peripheral trigeminal nerve(s) explaining the pain C. Onset within 6 months after the injury D. Associated with somatosensory symptoms and/or signs in the same neuroanatomically plausible distribution E. Not better accounted for by another ICOP or ICHD-3 diagnosis
Persistent dentoalveolar pain (PDAP)	ICOP Domain 6 Idiopathic	**Previously used terms:** Atypical odontalgia; primary persistent dentoalveolar pain disorder (PDAP); phantom tooth pain **Description:** Persistent unilateral intraoral dentoalveolar pain, rarely occurring in multiple sites, with variable features but recurring daily for more than 2 h per day for more than 3 months, in the absence of any preceding causative even **Diagnostic criteria:** A. Intraoral dentoalveolar pain fulfilling criteria B and C B. Recurring daily for >2 h/day for >3 months C. Pain has both of the following characteristics: 1. Localized to a dentoalveolar site (tooth or alveolar bone) 2. Deep, dull, pressure-like quality D. Clinical and radiographic examinations are normal, and local causes have been excluded E. Not better accounted for by another ICOP or ICHD-3 diagnosis

(continued)

Condition	Classification system	Diagnostic criteria
		ICHD https://www.ichd-3.org/how-to-use-the-classification/

Trigeminal Neuralgia	ICOP Domain 4 Neuropathic Classical trigeminal neuralgia (with neurovascular conflict); secondary TN and idiopathic TN	**Previously used term**: Tic douloureux
		Description: A disorder characterized by recurrent unilateral brief electric shock-like pains, abrupt in onset and termination, limited to the distribution of one or more divisions of the trigeminal nerve and triggered by innocuous stimuli. It may develop without apparent cause or be a result of another disorder. Additionally, there may or may not be concomitant continuous pain of moderate intensity within the affected division(s)
		Diagnostic criteria:
		A. Recurrent paroxysms of unilateral facial pain in the distribution(s) of one or more divisions of the trigeminal nerve, with no radiation beyond, and fulfilling criteria B and C
		B. The pain has all the following characteristics:
		  1. Lasting from a fraction of a second to 2 min
		  2. Severe intensity
		  3. Electric shock-like, shooting, stabbing or sharp in quality
		C. Precipitated by innocuous stimuli within the affected trigeminal distribution
		D. Not better accounted for by another ICOP or ICHD-3 diagnosis

Burning mouth syndrome	ICOP Domain 6 Idiopathic including BMS with somatosensory changes and BSM without somatosensory changes	**Previously used terms**: Stomatodynia; glossodynia (when confined to the tongue); primary burning mouth syndrome
		Description: An intraoral burning or dysaesthetic sensation, recurring daily for more than 2 h per day for more than 3 months, without evident causative lesions on clinical examination and investigation
		Diagnostic criteria:
		A. Oral pain fulfilling criteria B and C
		B. Recurring daily for >2 h per day for >3 months
		C. Pain has both of the following characteristics:
		  1. Burning quality
		  2. Felt superficially in the oral mucosa
		D. Oral mucosa is of normal appearance, and local or systemic causes have been excluded
		E. Not better accounted for by another ICOP or ICHD-3 diagnosis

prickling or pain described as shooting, stabbing, burning or having an electric shock sensations. Negative symptoms are described as diminished sensations due to loss of sensory function. Patients may also experience allodynia, hyperalgesia and anaesthesia dolorosa (pain in an area that is anaesthetic or numb) [43].

The diagnosis of NP is primarily based on patient history and physical examination. The Special interest Group on Neuropathic Pain (NeuPSIG) recently updated a grading system to assist with determining the level of certainty that the pain is neuropathic in nature and not related to other causes [44]. The grading system allows patients to be categorised into "possible", "probable" and "definite" NP [45].

Post-traumatic neuropathy (PTN) with pain: Over the last 10 years it has become evident that significant numbers of patients suffer from chronic pain as a result of routine surgery with over 30–40% of patients presenting in chronic pain, clinics being diagnosed with chronic postsurgical pain (CPSP) [11]. CPSP is known to be caused by a number of common surgical procedures for example; thoracotomy, breast surgery, limb amputation and herniorrhaphy. Within the trigeminal system, CPSP has been reported following local anaesthetic (LA) administration, dental extractions, endodontic procedures and dental implant placement. A study by Lobb and colleagues [46] found that most patients who suffered phantom tooth pain (chronic pain after dental surgery) did not revisit the dental surgeon. This does suggest that many dental surgeons will be underestimating the morbidity of the procedures.

PTN is difficult to diagnose as patients present without any clinically or radiographically demonstrable abnormality [45]. Neuropathic area may not be present and is currently an essential diagnostic criteria. Neuropathic pain in relation to dental implant placement is most commonly reported in the mandible; caused by traumatic injury to the inferior alveolar or lingual nerves, as a result of direct trauma from the drill or implant or ischaemia caused by swelling or haemorrhage [47]. To date, there have been only two published cases of CPSP in the maxilla following dental implant placement. However, there are many reports of painful post-traumatic trigeminal neuropathy. CPSP with neuropathic area within the trigeminal system is given many names (post-traumatic neuropathy, painful post-traumatic trigeminal neuropathy, persistent idiopathic dentoalveolar pain, atypical odontalgia). All these persistent postsurgical pain conditions may be attributable to chronic postsurgical pain; however, it is difficult to be conclusive without a demonstrable neuropathic area in relation to the previous surgery (post-traumatic neuropathic pain or persistent dentoalveolar pain disorder [PDAP II] diagnosis). The low incidence of CPSP in the trigeminal region may reflect the lack of central sensitisation due to most procedures being undertaken under LA [48].

Risk factors: Prevention of PTN with or without neuropathy may be possible and risk factors are becoming evident including:

- Preoperative screening of neuropathic pain, which does not respond to surgery or may worsen after surgery, is recommended. A high index of suspicion is required for the diagnosis of neuropathic pain as it can develop slowly over time. If neuropathic pain is suspected, a validated diagnostic screening tool such as the

Leeds Assessment of Neuropathic Symptoms and Signs (LANSS), the Self-reported LANSS (S-LANSS), the Neuropathic Pain Questionnaire (NPQ), the Douleur Neuropathique en 4 (DN4) questions, painDETECT and ID Pain may be useful. These verbal reports provide valuable information to the practitioner regarding pain quality: neuropathic pain is usually described as burning, painful, cold or electric shocks and may be associated with tingling, pins and needles, numbness or itching. These screening tools also serve as a good clinical record for follow-up post-treatment initiation, however, their sensitivity and specificity for the trigeminal system is poor [48].

- Pre-operative screening for specific patient factors known to increase risk including genetics (catecholamine-O-methyltransferase), preceding pain (intensity and chronicity), psychosocial factors (i.e. fear, memories, work, physical levels of activity, somatisation, anxiety, neuroticism, catastrophising and introversion), age (younger = increased risk breast surgery and herniorrhaphy/older = increased risk other surgery), gender (female = increased risk) [11].
- Preoperative medical screening: [11]
  - Raynaud's disease
  - Erythromelalgia
  - Irritable bowel syndrome
  - Migrainous headaches
  - Fibromyalgia

- Modifying surgery risk factors include the duration and extent of surgical procedure and technique (tension due to retraction) and high level perioperative reported pain levels. Prevention of chronic post-surgical pain may be possible [11] by using:
  - Multimodal management of severe acute postsurgical pain
  - Minimal access surgery
  - Intraoperative use of LA (international guidelines for prevention and management of post-operative chronic pain following inguinal hernia surgery)

The sensory examination includes; confirmation of a neuropathic area, a response to light touch, temperature, painful stimulus and vibration. Compare both sides and grade as normal, decreased or increased. Also, look for autonomic changes in colour, temperature, sweating and swelling.

Investigations: Haematology must be used to exclude systemic causes of neuropathy including; full blood count (FBC), erythrocyte sedimentation rate (ESR), glucose, creatinine, alanine transaminase (ALT), vitamin B12, serum protein immunoelectrophoresis and thyroid function. Assessing glycaemic control with an HbA1c is useful in patients who are diabetic. A glucose tolerance test may be helpful if the diabetic status is not known. Imaging may be required to exclude nerve damage usually with plane films and cone-beam computed tomography (CBCT) or magnetic resonance imaging (MRI) if a central lesion is suspected.

The pain that the patient is experiencing must be assessed on the functional and psychological impact. These must be managed alongside the pain using psychological interventions if the patient is amenable. The painful element or neuropathic pain due to neuropathy is sometimes considered to be of two types—neuralgic (sharp, stabbing pains as in TN) or neuropathic (altered sensations such as burning, tingling, "pins and needles") and so sometimes different treatments are given according to which type of pain is felt most often. Medical management of neuropathic pain [28], may include tricyclic antidepressants, gabapentin and/or pregabalin, topical drugs applied to the skin (LA or capsaicin) or Botoxin A injections where applicable. Surgery is indicated *urgently* for post-traumatic neuropathy related to wisdom teeth, implant or root canal surgery within 30 hours and rarely up to 3 months but not later.

Thus, chronic pain caused by surgery is a well-recognised phenomenon in the medical setting but remains mainly unrecognised and poorly diagnosed in dentistry. Fortunately, it is very rare in the trigeminal system, likely due to the regular use of LA injections [5]. In order for our profession to reliably develop evidence-based management of these conditions, alignment and rationalisation of the current nomenclature must be undertaken.

Management of a patient presenting with chronic postsurgical pain (PDAP II or PTN) should include:

- Referral to a clinical psychologist with an interest and experience in managing chronic orofacial pain patients for tailored Cognitive Behavioural Therapy.
- Referral to secondary care where medical management using either (1) Nortriptyline 10 mg nocte (increase to 40 mg over 4 weeks and wait at highest tolerated dose for 6 weeks to assess response) or 25 mg pregabalin nocte for 2 weeks and increase the dose over several months to 100 mg (50 mg mane and 50 mg nocte) can be provided.
- Referral to secondary care where Topical Versatis patches (2% lidocaine Grunenthal 12 h on 12 h off) cut out to cover the upper lip region and stuck to the skin using micropore can be provided for relief of elicited pain at night, thereby also preventing sleep interruption.

Mimicking dental pain: Elicited acute neuralgic pain to non-noxious stimuli (eating, tooth brushing, tooth tapping, cold) are features of PTN, and hence easily confused with various forms of toothache.

Trigeminal neuralgia (TN): Trigeminal neuralgia is the most frequent cranial neuralgia [6]. TN has been reported to be a rare disorder with reported incidences in the range of 4.5/100,000. There is a slight predilection towards females, and occurrence in the 50- to 70-year-old age group [49]. The elicited pain usually is spontaneous onset, occurs in V2 and V3 and is absent at night.

The aetiology and pathophysiology of TN have remained difficult to determine, although it is hypothesised that compression of the trigeminal root at or near the dorsal root entry zone by a blood vessel is a causative factor. Surgical data have consistently failed to provide high-quality data linking phenotype, MRI findings, operative findings and long-term outcome: therefore it is not possible to provide conclusive evidence that TN is caused solely by compression of the trigeminal nerve. A recent study using ultra-high-field MRI found high incidences of neurovascular compression in individuals (92%) with no symptoms of TN, and so suggests that there are other mechanisms involved [50].

There are three recognised types of trigeminal neuralgia (ICHD Beta 3): [13]

- Classical TN (purely paroxysmal or with concomitant continuous pain) TN with MRI proven vascular compression.
- Secondary TN (like other secondary neuropathies related to space-occupying lesion, multiple sclerosis [MS], Herpes Zoster or systemic disease).
- Idiopathic TN (purely paroxysmal or with concomitant continuous pain) no cause has been identified.

Presentation: Patients with trigeminal neuralgia experience facial pain limited to areas associated with one or more branches of the trigeminal nerve [2, 51]. The symptoms that patients experience are the result of compression of this nerve by vasculature or tumours. This type of pain can also be caused by demyelination in patients with MS. Pain attacks begin suddenly and last from several seconds to a couple of minutes. The pain is usually unilateral in nature and is described as sharp, shooting, shock-like, burning and excruciating. These attacks are usually accompanied by involuntary spasms or contractions of the facial muscles. Trigeminal neuralgia is usually triggered by non-painful physical stimulation of a specific area that is located close to the pain [6].

There is a substantial evidence base that carbamazepine (Tegretol) is the optimal medical drug of choice and most patients respond very quickly. However, there is a risk of Stephens Johnson syndrome reaction and neutropenia. If the patient is of Han Chinese origin the risk of adverse reaction is significant and genetic testing can be undertaken, but in many countries with a population at risk, the pragmatic step is to prescribe pregabalin. Microvascular decompression is also effective for patients where medication is problematic with adverse events of impact on the ability to work. This brain surgery has a morbidity risk of about 1%, depending on the patient, so is not a decision lightly undertaken.

Mimicking toothache: The elicited neuralgic pain on eating and brushing teeth Mimics cracked tooth, dentine hypersensitivity and reversible pulpitis. Differential factors include pain that is likely to be elicited by extraoral sites and a refractory period with cessation of elicited pain on continued stimulation. Treatment with carbamazepine (Tegretol) is usually effective. One of the most pressing issues is that preceding trigeminal neuralgia, there is increasing recognition of preTn or preTic is very likely to cause toothache-type symptoms in older patients. These older patients will have a highly restored dentition and dental teams will always find pathology on a dental radiograph if they try hard enough! The pain is episodic so the anti-inflammatory "test" will not work.

The clinician must reflect on the history presentation and non-response to routine care. They must take a step back and use the pain history to guide diagnosis rather than relying on investigations.

Other causes of secondary NP that may rarely mimic a toothache (see Table 3.4).

Table 3.4 Systemic factors contributing to ongoing chronic pain

Nutritional deficiencies
Fe, Ferritin, Zinc, Magnesium
Vit B complex, D, E
Malignancy exclude RED Flags
Compression by a space-occupying lesion centrally or peripherally NEOPLASIA
Metabolic Acromegaly, Hormonal neuropathy (Hypothyroidism, Diabetes), infarction (sickle cell hypoxic neural damage, giant cell arteritis)
Demyelination (Multiple sclerosis)
Infection Post viral neuropathy, Bacterial, Leprosy
Toxic Heavy metal poisoning (lead, mercury) radiation, thermal, chemotherapy, drugs
Auto immune problems: Lupus, Rheumatoid disease
Sarcoidosis and amyloidosis

Diabetic peripheral neuropathy is a condition that affects many patients with diabetes. In the United Kingdom, the annual incident rate per 10,000 population for painful diabetic neuropathy was 3.1. Diabetic neuropathy is recognised in patients with diabetes by the presence of peripheral nerve dysfunction symptoms after other causes have been excluded. Symptoms of this type of neuropathy include numbness, tingling, poor balance and pain that is described as burning, having electric shocks sensations and/or stabbing. Although the exact mechanism is unknown, this type of NP is thought to be the result of oxidative and inflammatory stress caused by metabolic dysfunction, which ultimately damages the nerve cells. Diabetic neuropathy plays a major role in foot ulcerations, the development of Charcot neuroarthropathy, falls and fractures [52].

HIV-associated peripheral sensory neuropathy (HIV-SN) is considered the most prevalent neurological complication associated with HIV infection. This type of neuropathy presents as a distal polyneuropathy in a symmetrical pattern that occurs in patients with both treated and untreated HIV infections. HIV-SN can be the result of injury to the nerve by the HIV itself, or it could be caused by medication-induced mitochondrial dysfunction of the nerve cells. Risk factors associated with the development of HIV-SN include exposure to neurotoxic antiretroviral drugs, increasing age, malnutrition, ethnicity, increasing height, certain genetic factors and comorbid conditions such as diabetes [53].

Chemotherapy-induced peripheral neuropathy (CIPN) is the most common neurological cancer treatment complication. It is a dose-dependent, adverse effect associated with chemotherapy agents such as platinum drugs, vinca alkaloids, bortezomib and taxanes. These agents cause sensory nerve damage in the dorsal root ganglion. Patients with CIPN describe the spectrum of pain and numbness as symmetric and distal, with a "glove and stocking" distribution. The symptoms may become progressively worse as chemotherapy is continued. In many cases, CIPN improves once the therapy is discontinued; however, with cisplatin and oxaliplatin, it may continue even after the drugs have been discontinued [54].

Postherpetic neuralgia (PHN) is NP that develops when the herpes zoster virus is reactivated. The virus remains latent in the dorsal root ganglion until the patient's immunocompetence begins to decrease due to increasing age, HIV infection, cancer or immunosuppressive therapy, at which time the virus can reactivate. The virus can affect the nerves through sensitisation (hyperexcitability) and deafferentation (sensory nerve death or damage). Pain is typically distributed unilaterally along spinal dermatomes or the ophthalmic branch of the trigeminal nerve. The annual incidence rate per 10,000 population for postherpetic neuralgia was 3.4 in the United Kingdom [55].

Burning mouth syndrome (BMS): Toothache is unlikely to be mimicked by BMS. Burning mouth syndrome (also known as stomatodynia) is an oral mucosal pain condition that is chronic, and absent of identifiable causative lesions, conditions or diseases. Reported prevalence in general populations varies from 1% to 15% according to diagnostic criteria, however, many studies include people with the symptom of burning mouth rather than true BMS as defined previously [56].

3.6   Idiopathic Pain

Persistent idiopathic facial pain (PIFP) and persistent idiopathic intraoral pain (PDAP) are chronic disorder recurring daily for more than 2 h per day over more than 3 months, in the absence of clinical neurological deficit. PIFP is the current terminology for atypical facial pain or atypical odonatlagia, and is characterised by daily or near daily pain that is initially confined but may subsequently spread. PIFP is often a difficult but important differential diagnosis among chronic facial pain syndromes. It has a continuous unchanging nature over many years despite many medical and surgical interventions [57].

Presentation: The pain is usually deep and poorly localised, and the quality is of burning, cramping or dull quality. The incidence is estimated as two to four per 100,000 but exact epidemiological data are lacking. Persistent idiopathic facial pain is a difficult diagnostic group compared to other pain categories and symptomatic causes must always be sought. The underlying pathophysiology is yet unknown and therapy is widely unspecific and ineffective [58].

Mimick toothache chronic orofacial pain PIFP is likely to be associated with patients presenting with multiple pain conditions or chronic widespread pain. Clinicians should be aware of patients presenting with a history of chronic widespread pain (CWP).

Chronic widespread pain (CWP): it is already recognised that the co-existence of headache further exacerbates clinical characteristics in patients with painful TMD, which implies the involvement of common mechanisms and pathways of vulnerability in these patients [59]. Up to 60% of patients with myalgic TMD present with co-existent headaches and considering all possible levels of interaction, a recommendation for multidisciplinary approaches by a team of OFP specialists and a neurologist (headache specialist) is important to attain the most precise differential diagnosis and initiate the best treatment [60].

Multidisciplinary care is essential in optimising patient safety, in OFP, by optimal diagnostics and early recognition of chronic pain, which improves the chances of successful management, and avoids frustration and disillusion both to patient and doctor. Another recommendation must include that education of dentists in primary headaches is essential and history taking should include headache history and migrainous and autonomic associated signs routinely questioned.

3.7   Conclusion

The complexity of the anatomy, neurobiological importance of the orofacial region and the variable presentation of toothache make potential pitfalls of diagnosis inevitable. These issues are compounded by the siloed training of clinicians providing often conflicting advice, or worse, undertaking unnecessary surgery, given to patients on their desperate journey to seek out a clear diagnosis and effective treatment of their OFP.

There is no 'dark art' in managing patients with COFP, using a holistic approach (Axis I and Axis II assessment) with key investigations when indicated. Clear communication will likely lead to identifying a diagnosis and there are clear guidelines for many of the pain presentations described (see Table 3.5).

Key lessons learned by the author from seeing many patients presenting with these chronic OFP conditions who often have experienced unnecessary medical, dental, ENT and other interventions include:

- Common things happen commonly, dental teams are likely to come across odontogenic pain rather than other complaints.

Table 3.5 Management of Orofacial Pain

Type of pain	Condition	Guidance	Medical management
Nociceptive pain	Dentine sensitivity	SDCEP prescribing guidance	Topical agents
Inflammatory pain	Irreversible pulpitis	SDCEP prescribing guidance	Extirpate RCT or extraction
	Dental abscess	FGDP AMS guidance	No antibiotics
Inflammatory pain ± mixed Ne centralised	TMD	TMD RDC guidance	Non interventional
	Arthromaylagia	FDS RCS TMD guidance	Analgesia Paracetamol
	Arthritides		ibroprufen Bite Guard
Neurovascular pain	Headaches migraine	NICE Guidance Adult headaches	TCAs, Triptans < GON Block or Botox
Neurovascular pain	Trigeminial Autonomic Cephalalgias	NICE Guidance Adult headaches	CH GON block SUNCT Lamotrogine PH indomethacin trial
Neuropathic pain	Primary PDAP 1 or post-traumatic	NICE neuropathic guidance adults	TCAs, Gabanoids, SSRIs
Neuropathic pain	Burning mouth syndrome	AAOP	TCAs, topical clonazepine, SSRIs
Centralised pain	PIFP Chronic headache	AAOP	TCAs, Gabanoids, SSRIs

- If the pain does not respond to anti-inflammatories (NSAIDs) then it is not inflammatory pain.
- If the patient's pain complaint is non-responsive to routine dental care, the clinician should re-evaluate rather than continuing unnecessary and possibly damaging treatment.
- Always ask the patient about coexisting pain conditions including chronic widespread pain, headaches and cervical spine pain.
- Be aware of the mental health comorbidity that may be driving the patient's suffering and behaviour.
- Always consider the chronology of the onset of pain and an event. It can be a non-physical life event that may predispose the patient to develop chronic pain. Conversely, pain related to a traumatic event may be neuropathic in nature.
- If the pain is complex or non-responsive to treatment, ask about site, onset, character, radiation, associated signs, timing, exacerbation and alleviating factors and severity—SOCRATES pain history, including migrainous and autonomic signs.
- There is increasing recognition of pre-Tn or pre-Tic preceding trigeminal neuralgia which is very likely to cause toothache-type symptoms in older patients. These older patients usually have a highly restored dentition and dental teams will commonly find pathology on a dental radiograph. It is wise to take a step back and use the pain history as a guide to diagnosis rather than relying on investigations.

References

1. Kalenderian E, Obadan-Udoh E, Maramaldi P, Etolue J, Yansane A, Stewart D, White J, Vaderhobli R, Kent K, Hebballi NB, Delattre V, Kahn M, Tokede O, Ramoni RB, Walji MF. Classifying adverse events in the dental office. J Patient Saf. 2017; https://doi.org/10.1097/PTS.0000000000000407. [Epub ahead of print].
2. Maramaldi P, Walji MF, White J, Etolue J, Kahn M, Vaderhobli R, Kwatra J, Delattre VF, Hebballi NB, Stewart D, Kent K, Yansane A, Ramoni RB, Kalenderian E. How dental team members describe adverse events. J Am Dent Assoc. 2016;147(10):803–11. https://doi.org/10.1016/j.adaj.2016.04.015. Epub 2016 Jun 3.
3. Hiivala N, Mussalo-Rauhamaa H. As the first symptom of oral cancer: a descriptive study. Oral Surg Oral Med Oral Pathol Oral Radiol Endod. 2006;102(1):56–61. Epub 2006 Apr 24.
4. Tefke HL, Murtomaa H. An analysis of dental patient safety incidents in a patient complaint and healthcare supervisory database in Finland. Acta Odontol Scand. 2016;74(2):81–9. https://doi.org/10.3109/00016357.2015.1042040. Epub 2015 May 13.
5. Lipton JA, Ship JA, Larach-Robinson D. Estimated prevalence and distribution of reported orofacial pain in the United States. J Am Dent Assoc. 1993;124(10):115–21.
6. Zakrzewska JM. Diagnosis and management of non-dental orofacial pain. Dent Update. 2007;34(3):134–6, 138–9.
7. May A, Svensson P. One nerve, three divisions, two professions and nearly no crosstalk? Cephalalgia. 2017;1:333102417704605. https://doi.org/10.1177/0333102417704605.
8. Cuffari L, Tesseroli de Siqueira JT, Nemr K, Rapaport A. Pain complaint as the first symptom of oral cancer: a descriptive study. Oral Surg Oral Med Oral Pathol Oral Radiol Endod. 2006;102(1):56–61. Epub 2006 Apr 24.
9. Woolf CJ. What is this thing called pain? J Clin Investig. 2010;120(11):3742–4.

10. Lewis C, Lynch H, Johnston B. Dental complaints in emergency departments: a national perspective. Ann Emerg Med. 2003;42(1):93–9.
11. Katz J, Seltzer Z. Transition from acute to chronic postsurgical pain: risk factors and protective factors. Expert Rev Neurother. 2009;9(5):723–44. https://doi.org/10.1586/ern.09.20.
12. International Headache Society (IHS). The international Classification of Headache Disorders. 3rd ed (beta version). Headache Classification Committee of the international Headache Society (IHS). First Published June 14. https://doi.org/10.1177/0333102413485658.
13. International Craniofacial Disorders Classification (ICHD 3). https://www.ichd-3.org/.
14. American Academy of Orofacial Pain (AAOP). http://www.aaop.org.
15. American Academy of Craniofacial Pain (AACP). https://www.aacfp.org/.
16. International Association for the international Study of Pain (IASP). Classification of chronic pain. 2nd ed (Revised). http://www.iasp-pain.org/PublicationsNews/Content.aspx? itemNumber=1673.
17. International Classification of Orofacial Pain, 1st edition (ICOP), Cephalalgia. 2020;40(2):129–221. https://doi.org/10.1177/0333102419893823. PMID: 32103673.
18. Desrosiers M, Evans GA, Keith PK, Wright ED, Kaplan A, Bouchard J, Ciavarella A, Doyle PW, Javer AR, Leith ES, Mukherji A, Schellenberg RR, Small P, Witterick IJ. Canadian clinical practice guidelines for acute and chronic rhinosinusitis. Allergy Asthma Clin Immunol. 2011;7(1):2.
19. Eross E, Dodick DO, Eross M. Headache 2007. Prevalence of facial pain in migraine is also reported. Cephalgia. 2009;30:92–6.
20. Lipton RB, et al. Migraine diagnosis and treatment: results from the American Migraine Study II. Headache. 2001;41(7):638–45.
21. Schreiber CP, Hutchinson S, Webster CJ, Ames M, Richardson MS, Powers C. Prevalence of migraine in patients with a history of self-reported or physician-diagnosed "sinus". Headache. Arch Intern Med. 2004;164(16):1769–72.
22. Graff-Radford SB. Facial pain, cervical pain, and headache. Continuum. 2012;18(4): 869–82.
23. Travell JG, Simons DG. Myofascial pain and disfunction: the trigger point manual. 1st ed. Baltimore: Williams and Wilkins; 1983.
24. de Oliveira Franco AC, de Siqueira JT, Mansur AJ. Bilateral facial pain from cardiac origin. A case report. Br Dent J. 2005;198:679–80.
25. Kreiner M, Okessn J. Toothache of cardiac origin. J Orofac Pain. 1999;13:201–7.
26. Lopez-Lopez J, Jane-Salas LG-VE, Estrugo-Devesa A, ChimenosKüstner E, Roca-Elias J. Orofacial pain of cardiac origin: review literature and clinical cases. Med Oral Patol Oral Cir Bucal. 2012;17(4):e538–44.
27. Rothwell PM. Angina and myocardial infarction presenting with pain confined to the ear. Postgrad Med J. 1993;69:300–1.
28. Hayashi B, Maeda M, Tsuruoka M, Inoue T. Neural mechanisms that underlie angina-induced referred pain in the trigeminal nerve territory: a c-Fos study in rats. ISRN Pain. 2013;2013:671503. https://doi.org/10.1155/2013/671503. eCollection 2013.
29. Wong JK, Wood RE, McLean M. Pain preceding recurrent head and neck cancer. J Orofac Pain. 1998;12(1):52–9.
30. Simard EP, Ward EM, Siegel R, Jemal A. Cancers with increasing incidence trends in the United States: 1999 through 2008. CA Cancer J Clin. 2012;62(4):277. Article first published online: 1 May 2012.
31. Schiffman E, Ohrbach R, Truelove E, Look J, Anderson G, Goulet JP, List T, Svensson P, Gonzalez Y, Lobbezoo F, Michelotti A, Brooks SL, Ceusters W, Drangsholt M, Ettlin D, Gaul C, Goldberg LJ, Haythornthwaite JA, Hollender L, Jensen R, John MT, De Laat A, de Leeuw R, Maixner W, van der Meulen M, Murray GM, Nixdorf DR, Palla S, Petersson A, Pionchon P, Smith B, Visscher CM, Zakrzewska J, Dworkin SF, International RDC/TMD Consortium Network, International Association for Dental Research; Orofacial Pain Special Interest Group, International Association for the Study of Pain. Diagnostic Criteria for Temporomandibular

Disorders (DC/TMD) for clinical and research applications: recommendations of the international RDC/TMD Consortium Network* and Orofacial Pain Special Interest Group. J Oral Facial Pain Headache. 2014;28(1):6–27. https://doi.org/10.11607/jop.1151.

32. Wright EF. Referred craniofacial pain patterns in patients with temporomandibular disorder. J Am Dent Assoc. 2000;131(9):1307–15.

33. Lim PF, Maixner W, Khan AA. Temporomandibular disorder and comorbid pain conditions. J Am Dent Assoc. 2011;142(12):1365–7.

34. Yoon MS, Mueller D, Hansen N, Poitz F, Slomke M, Dommes P, Diener HC, Katsarava Z, Obermann M. Prevalence of facial pain in migraine: a population-based study. Cephalalgia. 2010;30(1):92–6. https://doi.org/10.1111/j.1468-2982.2009.01899.x.

35. Hussain A, Stiles MA, Oshinsky ML. Pain remapping in migraine: a novel characteristic following trigeminal nerve injury. Headache. 2010;50(4):669–71.

36. Obermann M, Mueller D, Yoon MS, Pageler L, Diener H, Katsarava Z. Migraine with isolated facial pain: a diagnostic challenge. Cephalalgia. 2007;27(11):1278–82. Epub 2007 Sep 10.

37. Nixdorf DR, Velly AM, Alonso AA. Neurovascular pains: implications of migraine for the oral and maxillofacial surgeon. Oral Maxillofac Surg Clin North Am. 2008;20(2):221–35, vi–vii. https://doi.org/10.1016/j.coms.2007.12.008.

38. Kelman L. Migraine pain location: a tertiary care study of 1283 migraineurs. Headache. 2005;45:1038–47.

39. Noma N, Shimizu K, Watanabe K, Young A, Imamura Y, Khan J. Cracked tooth syndrome mimicking trigeminal autonomic cephalalgia: a report of four cases. Quintessence Int. 2017;48(4):329–37. https://doi.org/10.3290/j.qi.a37688.

40. Wei DY, Yuan Ong JJ, Goadsby PJ. Overview of trigeminal autonomic cephalalgias: nosologic evolution, diagnosis, and management. Ann Indian Acad Neurol. 2018;21(Suppl 1):S39–44.

41. Benoliel R, Sharav Y, Haviv Y, Almoznino G. Tic, triggering, and tearing: from CTN to SUNHA. Headache. 2017;57(6):997–1009.

42. Meacham K, Shepherd A, Mohapatra D, et al. Neuropathic pain: central vs peripheral mechanisms. Curr Pain Headache Rep. 2017;21(6):28. https://doi.org/10.1007/s11916-017-0629-5.

43. Jensen T, Baron R, Haanpää M, et al. A new definition of neuropathic pain. Pain. 2011;152(10):2204–5. https://doi.org/10.1016/j.pain.2011.06.017.

44. Mohapatra D, et al. Neuropathic pain: central vs peripheral mechanisms. Curr Pain Headache Rep. 2017;21(6):28. https://doi.org/10.1007/s11916-017-0629-5.

45. Finnerup N, Haroutounian S, Kamerman P, et al. Neuropathic pain: an updated grading system for research and clinical practice. Pain. 2016;157(8):1599–606. https://doi.org/10.1097/j.pain.0000000000000492.

46. Renton T. Minimising and managing nerve injuries in dental surgical procedures. Faculty Dental J. 2011;2(4):164–71.

47. Renton T. Oral surgery: Part 4. Minimising and managing nerve injuries and other complications. Br Dent J. 2013;215(8):393–9. https://doi.org/10.1038/sj.bdj.2013.993. Review.

48. Baad-Hansen L, Benoliel R. Neuropathic orofacial pain: facts and fiction. Cephalalgia. 2017;37(7):670–9.

49. Hall GC, Carroll D, Parry D, McQuay HJ. Epidemiology and treatment of neuropathic pain: the UK primary care perspective. Pain. 2006;122(1–2):156–62.

50. Peker S, Dincer A, Necmettin Pamir M. Vascular compression of the trigeminal nerve is a frequent finding in asymptomatic individuals: 3-T MR imaging of 200 trigeminal nerves using 3D CISS sequences. Acta Neurochir. 2009;151(9):1081–8.

51. Selby G, Lance JW. Observations on 500 cases of migraine and allied vascular headache. J Neurol Neurosurg Psychiatry. 1960;23:23–32.

52. Pop-Busui R, Boulton A, Feldman E, et al. Diabetic neuropathy: a position statement by the American Diabetes Association. Diabetes Care. 2017;40(1):136–54. https://doi.org/10.2337/dc16-2042.

53. Woldeamanuel Y, Kamerman P, Veliotes D, et al. Development, validation, and field-testing of an instrument for clinical assessment of HIV-associated neuropathy and neuropathic pain

in resource-restricted and large population study settings. PLoS One. 2016;11(10):e0164994. https://doi.org/10.1371/journal.pone.0164994.

54. Esin E, Yalcin S. Neuropathic cancer pain: what we are dealing with? How to manage it? Onco Targets Ther. 2014;7:599–618.

55. Hershman DL, Lacchetti C, Dworkin RH, et al. Prevention and management of chemotherapy-induced peripheral neuropathy in survivors of adult cancers: American Society of Clinical Oncology clinical practice guideline. J Clin Oncol. 2014;32(18):1941–67. https://doi.org/10.1200/JCO.2013.54.0914.

56. Woda A, Grushka M. Burning mouth syndrome. In: Zakrzewska JM, editor. Orofacial pain. 1st ed. Oxford, UK: Oxford University Press; 2009. p. 83–92.

57. Weiss AL, Ehrhardt KP, Tolba R. Atypical facial pain: a comprehensive, evidence-based review. Curr Pain Headache Rep. 2017;21(2):8. https://doi.org/10.1007/s11916-017-0609-9.

58. Baad-Hansen L. Atypical odontalgia - pathophysiology and clinical management. J Oral Rehabil. 2008;35(1):1–11.

59. Costa YM, Alves da Costa DR, de Lima Ferreira AP, Porporatti AL, Svensson P, Rodrigues Conti PC, Bonjardim LR. Headache exacerbates pain characteristics in temporomandibular disorders. J Oral Facial Pain Headache. 2017;31(4):339–45.

60. Conti PC, Costa YM, Goncalves DA, Svensson P. Headaches and myofascial temporomandibular disorders: overlapping entities, separate managements? J Oral Rehabil. 2016;43(9):702–15.

Psychological Theories of Pain

4

Chris Penlington, Monika Urbanek, and Sarah Barker

Learning Objectives

- To explain the limitations of the medical model of care when working with persistent orofacial pain.
- To understand how the application of psychological theory to persistent pain has developed over time.
- To describe contemporary psychological theories of pain.

Traditionally dental treatment has tended to be underpinned by the medical model of care, which assumes that symptoms such as pain are caused by an underlying disease process or physical damage. According to the medical model, symptoms are likely to resolve once, all relevant underlying causes are effectively treated. However, research studies have shown that the relationship between pain and observable tissue pathology is relatively weak [1]. Everyday experiences of pain may include occurrences that could not be explained by the medical model.

It is common for people to experience the sensation of pain without underlying disease process or physical damage, e.g. when first getting into a hot bath with cold feet and to experience continuing damage without pain e.g. a week after breaking an arm or leg before the injury is fully healed. Clinical experience, both in dentistry and the wider field of pain management includes cases where no direct link can be

C. Penlington (✉)
School of Dental Sciences, Newcastle University, Newcastle upon Tyne, UK
e-mail: Chris.Penlington@newcastle.ac.uk

M. Urbanek
Croydon Health Services NHS Trust, Croydon, UK
e-mail: monikaurbanek@nhs.net

S. Barker
Private Practice, London, UK

© The Author(s), under exclusive license to Springer Nature Switzerland AG 2022   49
T. Renton (ed.), *Optimal Pain Management for the Dental Team*, BDJ Clinician's
Guides, https://doi.org/10.1007/978-3-030-86634-1_4

observed between physical disease or damage and the experience of pain. Persistent orofacial pain (POFP) conditions, where pain often continues despite the absence of objective physical findings, are an example of this.

4.1 History of Psychological Approaches to Pain Management

An emerging awareness of such instances has prompted a shift towards a multidimensional view of pain. Such a view acknowledges a broad range of pain drivers which include biological, psychological and social factors [2].

4.1.1 Gate Control Theory

The first milestone towards this understanding was the publication of the seminal gate control theory of pain in 1965 [3]. The Gate control theory proposed that messages from the body converge on the dorsal horns of the spinal cord and the brain, where they were combined with other information to determine the neural response and thus the experience of pain. The dorsal horns of the spinal cord were conceptualised as being like a "gate", which may open or close to signals from the body depending on a range of factors including past experience, attention or cognitive variables Thus the gate-control theory introduced the concept that pain can be influenced by top-down processing by the brain which can attenuate or intensify pain using a variety of mechanisms depending on contextual factors in the environment.

The Gate control theory provided a potential explanation for how pain might vary in response to a range of factors. Related to this is the question of why pain might vary in this way. This question was also addressed by Patrick Wall [4], who proposed that pain is not in fact an indicator of tissue damage or disease. Rather, like hunger or thirst, it is a motivational state that functions primarily to guide behaviour. That is to say that, just as thirst may motivate the behaviour of drinking, pain may serve to shape behaviour towards rest and recuperation. Taking this kind of functional perspective, it is easier to understand how in one context a severe injury could be painless (for example during battle when survival depends on continuing to fight) whereas in another a relatively minor occurrence could result in a high level of pain (for example a migraine triggered by stress).

4.1.2 The Neuromatrix

In the light of the above understanding and of scientific advances in the neuroscience of pain, Melzack and Wall published the neuromatrix theory of pain [5]. The neuromatrix theory proposes a body-self neuromatrix, which triggers various output patterns or "neurosignatures" in response to multiple influences. These patterns are widely distributed throughout the cerebral cortex and can trigger behavioural programs for post-injury, disease or chronic stress [5]. Thus this theory brings together potential pain mechanisms along with their functional relevance and accounts for advancing understanding in the field of neuroscience.

Importantly, the neuromatrix theory proposes that pain neurosignatures can be triggered even without sensory input from the periphery, that the neuromatrix is the primary mechanism for generating the neural pattern that produces pain and that this itself can trigger perceptual, homeostatic and behavioural mechanisms of response [5]. It can therefore account for some of the signs that frequently accompany pain including redness, swelling and tenderness, which may be seen as a physiological response to the threat of damage in some cases.

4.2   Psychological Theories

The publication of the Gate control theory marked the beginning of a shift in the understanding of pain away from a purely mechanical conceptualisation and towards a multidimensional experience affected by a range of biological, psychological and social factors. Alongside this shifting understanding came the possibility of applying psychological principles to the treatment of long-term pain.

4.2.1   Behavioural Approach

Traditionally, behavioural approaches were being used to treat mental health problems such as fear and phobias with some success [6]. The behavioural approach was applied to the management of pain by Wilbert Fordyce [7], leading to the establishment of pain clinics that incorporated psychological science into the management of pain [8]. Behavioural therapy applied the principles of behavioural conditioning to pain behaviours, aiming to use operant conditioning techniques to increase healthy behaviours and reduce pain behaviour.

Operant conditioning refers to the systematic application of specified consequences to behaviour, which influences the likelihood of the behaviour being repeated. Behaviour can be reinforced by positive (where the behaviour is followed by a rewarding consequence) or negative (where the behaviour is followed by a consequence which is also rewarding, due to the cessation of an unpleasant experience) reinforcement and will be more likely to recur. On the other hand, behaviour can be reduced if it is followed by extinction (no consequence) or punishment (an unpleasant consequence). Behavioural therapy involves using these contingencies in a systematic way to strengthen adaptive behaviours such as active engagement in meaningful activities and to weaken behaviours seen as problematic ie excessive resting or complaining. Within this protocol relaxation skills were also taught and applied alongside graded exposure to systematically desensitise patients to an increasing range of activities. An important part of behavioural protocols is the need for a careful "functional analysis" of behaviours and consequences which need to be considered on an individual basis since something that is experienced as rewarding to one person may be regarded as unpleasant by another. Many of the behavioural innovations employed by Fordyce remain relevant today, including the consideration of pain behaviours as targets of treatment and the need for individual functional analyses. Behavioural therapy for pain also introduced the assertion that precipitating and maintaining factors to a problem are often quite different, which also remains highly relevant to current practice.

4.2.2 Cognitive Approach

The behavioural approach focused on behaviour, which could be objectively observed. It did not take account of non-observable phenomena such as emotions and thoughts. Within clinical psychology in general the recognition and impact of thoughts and thinking patterns [9] received increasing attention through the 1970s and 1980s, leading to the development of cognitive therapy, an approach that puts much more emphasis on internal, unobservable events including thoughts and beliefs. This approach came to be known as "second wave" behavioural therapy and approaches focusing on changing observable behaviour through classical and operant conditioning became known as the "first wave".

Within multidisciplinary pain clinics, cognitive and behavioural approaches were naturally combined into Cognitive-Behavioural therapy (CBT) [8], an approach which, again, mirrored wider developments within clinical psychology. Cognitive-behavioural theories of pain are based on the premise that thoughts, emotions, behaviours and physical sensations are all interrelated and exist within a particular context that is also influential. Small changes in any of these areas can have wide-ranging influences through the circular effect of their influence on each of the areas. The CBT model is often presented diagrammatically and illustrates how, within a particular person, the different areas of the model may link with each other and create "vicious cycles" which can increase symptomatic distress. An example of such a cycle is illustrated in Fig. 4.1.

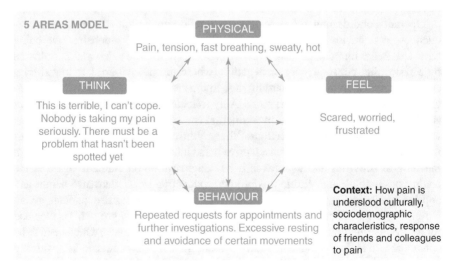

Fig. 4.1 An example of a cognitive behavioural formulation of persistent pain

Having identified thoughts or behaviours which are thought to feed into cycles in this way, psychological therapists will then work collaboratively with patients employing a variety of techniques to address potential issues and reverse vicious cycles.

4.2.3   Thoughts and Beliefs

A significant body of research has focused on identifying specific thoughts or beliefs, which may be implicated in poor outcomes in persistent pain and could potentially be modified with CBT. In terms of cognitive processes, research has highlighted a relationship between pain-related beliefs and appraisals with pain intensity, depression, physical disability, activity and social role limitations [10]. Pain catastrophising can be described as the magnification of the threat of, rumination about and perceived inability to cope with pain [11]. It has been found to be associated with greater physical and psychosocial dysfunction even after controlling for pain and depression levels [12]. Fear-avoidance which refers to activity avoidance due to fear of increased pain or bodily harm has also been shown to be important in pain and physical and psychosocial function [10, 13]. Self-efficacy beliefs, which refer to the confidence a person has that they can engage in behaviour, which will make a difference to their situation, have also been identified as important [14].

The theory behind cognitive behavioural therapy of pain would suggest that if such beliefs could be identified and changed, the pain would then be likely to have a lesser impact on mood, quality of life and disability. In a study of CBT for patients with temporomandibular disorders (TMD), such mediation effects were indeed reported for beliefs about pain, catastrophisation and self-efficacy [15]. However, another study has failed to replicate these findings [16]. It remains unclear therefore whether the targeted treatment that achieves changes in cognitive behaviour translates into the improvements that are seen following CBT in outcome measures.

4.2.4   Physical Sensations

The experience of persistent pain includes physical sensations of the pain itself and is also related to an individual's response to this pain. Injury and pain typically trigger the "fight or flight" response. This response is the body's way of dealing with immediate threats and is mediated by the autonomic nervous system and the hormonal system [17]. Persistent pain is often associated with an increase in anxiety and agitation, which can manifest as a strong drive to seek medical help and find a cure [18]. A dilemma for the chronic pain patient is that the pain constitutes a persistent and inescapable source of threat. This can lead to hypervigilance. The findings published by Dehghani et al. [19] show that chronic pain patients selectively attend to sensory aspects of pain. This felt a sense of threat could function as a maintaining factor for pain in terms of the neuromatrix and could be heightened not just by continuing pain but also beliefs that this is linked to damage and that therefore the problem is not being taken seriously by treatment providers. This would be addressed within CBT by aiming to address a patient's beliefs and understanding about pain and provide appropriate pain education.

4.2.5 Behaviours

The CBT model also suggests that coping skills are important as constant pain could overwhelm a person's ability to cope using their usual strategies [20]. A range of skills is often taught including relaxation, activity management and planning, and specific exercises. Again, however, there is little evidence to link engagement with such skills to outcome following pain management interventions [21, 22]. Whereas CBT has been associated with good outcomes for pain management, including persistent orofacial pain [23], mechanisms behind this improvement remain unclear.

4.2.6 Third Wave Approaches

Second-wave cognitive behavioural therapies have tended to focus on the content of thoughts and on helping people to rationally challenge thoughts, which are seen as "dysfunctional" or "irrational" and which may perpetuate psychological distress. For example, the thought "I can't cope with this pain" might be addressed in a systematic way by writing down evidence of times when the person has successfully managed to cope with similar levels of pain along with education about how thoughts can sometimes be inaccurate and ideas for new techniques that they could explore. Within this model, changing thoughts are seen as key to more adaptive functioning.

However, worrying thoughts about ongoing and intense pain may not be unrealistic. McCracken and Eccelston [24] found that worries about pain typically fell into one of four categories, elaborated here with possible examples from orofacial pain:

1. **Pain experience**
      (e.g. this pain just keeps hurting)
2. **Disability**
      (e.g. I can't have conversations like I used to)
3. **Medical uncertainty**
      (e.g. have I got a new infection in my tooth?)
4. **Negative effect**
      (e.g. I'm weak for not stopping the procedure).

It was shown that worry in chronic pain differs from generalised anxiety disorder (GAD), and is a normal response to the abnormal situation of chronic pain [24]. McCracken and Eccleston went on to suggest that acceptance of chronic pain was correlated with less pain, reduced disability, less pain-related anxiety, higher levels of daily activities and better employment opportunities [24].

The construct of acceptance is relevant to a group of approaches including acceptance and commitment therapy (ACT) and mindfulness-based interventions (MBis), known as "third wave" CBT. At the heart of such interventions is the theoretical construct of "psychological flexibility" and its opposite, "experiential avoidance" [25]. The term "psychological flexibility" refers to the capacity and willingness to remain in contact with present moment experience, even when it is difficult or unpleasant. Experiential avoidance on the other hand refers to an unwillingness to remain connected to certain internal experiences including thoughts, feelings and physical sensations that are painful or uncomfortable. ACT is based on the theory that attempts to avoid pain and other difficult internal experiences have the unintended consequence of restricting engagement in activities that are personally meaningful and important. Overall, this restriction is considered to be linked with poor outcomes such as increased disability.

Research into the mechanisms behind third-wave approaches has been more fruitful than in traditional CBT. For example, Eifert and Heffner [26] compared the effects of acceptance versus control strategies applied to aversive interoceptive stimulation, and found that those using acceptance-based strategies had less catastrophic thoughts, and less intense fear and cognitive symptoms. Feldner et al. [27] demonstrated that those who used experiential avoidance as a way of coping with an aversive cold-pressor task had lower levels of pain endurance and tolerance. Costa and Pinto-Gouvia [28] conducted hierarchical regression analyses, and showed that experiential avoidance and self-compassion are the factors that mostly explain psychological distress. In their discussion, they suggested that when people with chronic pain are willing to remain in contact with particular private experiences rather than attempting to control them, they reported less depression, anxiety and stress. Branstetter-Rost et al. [29] evaluated the effect of adding in a personalised values-based exercise in an acceptance-based treatment for pain and found that helping patients to clarify the values that are important to them in life makes a significant contribution to treatment.

An alternative method of researching relevant processes of change is to link what people do, or pain outcomes to measures of neural activity. Zeidan et al. [30, 31] have reviewed research into meditation practices including mindfulness, which aims to illuminate neural pathways through which these practices may modulate pain. Initial findings were reported to suggest that improvements in pain in novice meditators might be supported by frequent cognitive re-appraisal through the practice of focused attention. For these people reductions in pain were accompanied by increased activation in the orbitofrontal cortex (OFC). By contrast, in experienced meditators, reductions in pain were associated with reduced activity in the OFC which the authors suggested may reflect the shift with increased meditative experience from cognitive reappraisal towards a more appraisal-free state and from focused attention to open meditation [31]. This appraisal-free state could be interpreted as a state of psychological flexibility since it involves allowing present moment experience to be just as it is without attempts to change or avoid it. Recent research by Zeidan et al. [32] has also described neural correlates of dispositional mindfulness, which has been found to be related to reduced pain in response to a noxious heat stimulus. These studies have the potential to link a theoretical model to neural mechanisms leading to a greater understanding of proposed mechanisms of change which perhaps, in the future could be more fully understood and targeted by a more diverse range of treatment approaches than is currently available.

4.3   Focus of Therapy

One challenge to incorporating psychological theory within the field of persistent pain has been that, within a wider medical culture that tends to emphasise physical or biological changes, the incorporation of a psychological angle can be seen as dismissive, suggesting that the pain is "not real" or "in the head". This is in fact a common misconception about the implications of engaging in psychological work and can present a major barrier to engagement. Psychologists have tended to respond to patient concerns about being labelled in this way by stressing the huge impact that pain has on various aspects of life and focusing on how psychological interventions can help in this area.

This approach has the advantage of reducing the risk that patients will feel disbelieved. Moreover, neither the neuromatrix nor the biopsychosocial model includes explicit theories of how psychological and social factors specifically interact to influence pain, and research into potential mechanisms for this remains at an early stage. It makes sense therefore that psychological interventions including cognitive behavioural therapy (CBT) and acceptance and commitment therapy (ACT) emphasise that pain reduction is not a primary target of treatment. This rationale discourages an overt focus on pain, something which otherwise may lead to pain magnification. It also supports patients to focus outwards and consider their life within a wider perspective, enabling them to consider changes that are within their control and likely to lead to general improvements in their life whether or not pain can be reduced. An alternative approach focuses on providing pain education explicitly to reduce the sense of threat that may be experienced with persistent pain [33]. The "explain pain" (EP) approach consists of employing a range of educational methods and resources which aim to shift patients' understanding of pain from that of being an indication of tissue damage or disease towards representing a perceived need to protect body tissue [33]. Perhaps building on EP, pain neuroscience education is gaining credibility as an effective way of addressing persistent pain [34]. Educational material, which is often tailored to the individual, aims to reduce misconceptions and, therefore, fear about the pain which otherwise can act directly and indirectly as powerful drivers of the perceived threat and of continuing pain. A newer approach, cognitive functional therapy (CFT), developed as a treatment for back pain also provides tailored education about pain and how it works while explicitly linking this to strategies for movement and everyday activities [35]. Like CBT and ACT, both of these interventions are firmly rooted within a biopsychosocial framework and target a range of factors that according to a biopsychosocial understanding of pain, may be relevant to the maintenance of the pain state.

The above approaches, which clearly integrate a psychological understanding of pain as a major treatment component, differ from more traditional psychological approaches to pain management in that they explicitly target a reduction in pain as a primary outcome in addition to secondary outcomes of improved mood and ability to engage in valued life activities. They repeatedly return to a core functional understanding of pain. Within a pain functional approach, pain is understood as an output associated with felt danger or threat; it, therefore, follows that reducing the threat (which is achieved with targeted education about pain and about the impact of strategies for pain control which may lead to long-term exacerbations) can reduce pain. Compassion-focused therapy, which uses a range of methods to reduce threat-based emotions such as shame also shows promise for pain management [36] and could also be seen as relevant within this philosophy.

Research has been lacking, to date, in psychological approaches to POFP guided by a functional understanding of pain. Such an approach may be a good fit for the population, particularly in the light of recently published guidelines for the treatment of TMD [37] which stress the importance of education and reduction of parafunctional activities and advise that pain resolution is likely for patients who actively self-manage.

4.4 Summary

There is compelling evidence that pain is a complex and multifactorial experience. While biological factors such as damage and infection are strong drivers of pain in many cases, both theory and evidence point to the importance of a range of psychological and social factors in the experience of pain. Such an understanding opens up the potential for a broader range of treatment targets and approaches. Most interventions for POFP will benefit from integrating an understanding of psychological and social factors. However, at present, the theories that inform such interventions warrant further research and remain incomplete.

References

1. Brinjikji W, Luetmer PH, Comstock B, Bresnahan BW, Chen L, Deyo R, et al. Systematic literature review of imaging features of spinal degeneration in asymptomatic populations. Am J Neuroradiol. 2015;36(4):811–6.
2. Ehde DM, Dillworth TM, Turner JA. Cognitive-behavioral therapy for individuals with chronic pain: efficacy, innovations, and directions for research. Am Psychol. 2014;69(2):153.
3. Melzack R, Wall PD. Pain mechanisms: a new theory. Science. 1965;150(3699):971–9.
4. Wall PD. On the relation of injury to pain the John J. Bonica Lecture. Pain. 1979;6(3):253–64.
5. Melzack R. From the gate to the neuromatrix. Pain. 1999;82:S121–S6.
6. Wolpe J. Psychotherapy by reciprocal inhibition. Cond Reflex. 1968;3(4):234–40.
7. Fordyce WE, Fowler RS, Lehmann JF, Delateur BJ. Some implications of learning in problems of chronic pain. J Chronic Dis. 1968;21(3):179–90.
8. Gatchel RJ. Perspectives on pain: a historical overview. Psychosocial factors in pain: critical perspectives. New York: The Guilford Press; 1999. p. 3–17.
9. Beck AT. Cognitive therapy: nature and relation to behavior therapy. Behav Ther. 1970;1(2):184–200.
10. Gatchel RJ, Peng YB, Peters ML, Fuchs PN, Turk DC. The biopsychosocial approach to chronic pain: scientific advances and future directions. Psychol Bull. 2007;133(4):581.
11. Edwards RR, Cahalan C, Mensing G, Smith M, Haythornthwaite JA. Pain, catastrophizing, and depression in the rheumatic diseases. Nat Rev Rheumatol. 2011;7(4):216.
12. Velly AM, Look JO, Carlson C, Lenton PA, Kang W, Holcroft CA, et al. The effect of catastrophizing and depression on chronic pain-a prospective cohort study of temporomandibular muscle and joint pain disorders. Pain. 2011;152(10):2377–83.

13. Leeuw M, Goossens ME, Linton SJ, Crombez G, Boersma K, Vlaeyen JW. The fear-avoidance model of musculoskeletal pain: current state of scientific evidence. J Behav Med. 2007;30(1):77–94.
14. Litt MD, Porto FB. Determinants of pain treatment response and nonresponse: identification of TMD patient subgroups. J Pain. 2013;14(11):1502–13.
15. Turner JA, Holtzman S, Mancl L. Mediators, moderators, and predictors of therapeutic change in cognitive-behavioral therapy for chronic pain. Pain. 2007;127(3):276–86.
16. McCracken LM, MacKichan F, Eccleston C. Contextual cognitive-behavioral therapy for severely disabled chronic pain sufferers: effectiveness and clinically significant change. Eur J Pain. 2007;11(3):314–22.
17. Hall JE. Guyton and Hall textbook of medical physiology e-book. Amsterdam: Elsevier Health Sciences; 2010.
18. Van Griensven H, Barker S, Galindo H. Pain in practice: theory and treatment strategies for manual therapists. Amsterdam: Elsevier Health Sciences; 2005.
19. Dehghani M, Sharpe L, Nicholas M. Modification of attentional biases in chronic pain patients: a preliminary study. Eur J Pain. 2004;8(6):585–94.
20. Turk DC, Meichenbaum D, Genest M. Pain and behavioral medicine: a cognitive-behavioral perspective. New York: Guilford Press; 1983.
21. Kotiranta U, Suvinen T, Forssell H. Tailored treatments in temporomandibular disorders: where are we now? A systematic qualitative literature review. J Oral Facial Pain Headache. 2014;28(1):28–37.
22. Wig AD, Aaron LA, Turner JA, Huggins KH, Truelove E. Short-term clinical outcomes and patient compliance with temporomandibular disorder treatment recommendations. J Orofacial Pain. 2004;18(3):203–13.
23. Turner JARJM. Cognitive-behavioral therapy for chronic pain. In: Loeser JDBJJ, editor. Bonica's management of pain. 3rd ed. Philadelphia, PA: Lippincott Williams & Wilkins; 2001. p. 1751–8.
24. McCracken LM, Eccleston C. Coping or acceptance: what to do about chronic pain? Pain. 2003;105(1–2):197–204.
25. Hayes SC, Luoma JB, Bond FW, Masuda A, Lillis J. Acceptance and commitment therapy: model, processes and outcomes. Behav Res Ther. 2006;44(1):1–25.
26. Eifert GH, Heffner M. The effects of acceptance versus control contexts on avoidance of panic-related symptoms. J Behav Ther Exp Psychiatry. 2003;34(3–4):293–312.
27. Feldner MT, Hekmat H, Zvolensky MJ, Vowles KE, Secrist Z, Leen-Feldner EW. The role of experiential avoidance in acute pain tolerance: a laboratory test. J Behav Ther Exp Psychiatry. 2006;37(2):146–58.
28. Costa J, Pinto Gouveia J. Experiential avoidance and self compassion in chronic pain. J Appl Soc Psychol. 2013;43(8):1578–91.
29. Branstetter-Rost A, Cushing C, Douleh T. Personal values and pain tolerance: does a values intervention add to acceptance? J Pain. 2009;10(8):887–92.
30. Zeidan F. Brain mechanisms supporting the modulation of pain by mindfulness meditation. J Neurosci. 2011;31(14):5540.
31. Zeidan F, Grant JA, Brown CA, McHaffie JG, Coghill RC. Mindfulness meditation-related pain relief: evidence for unique brain mechanisms in the regulation of pain. Neurosci Lett. 2012;520(2):165–73.
32. Zeidan F, Salomons T, Farris SR, Emerson NM, Adler-Neal A, Jung Y, et al. Neural mechanisms supporting the relationship between dispositional mindfulness and pain. Pain. 2018;159(12):2477–85.
33. Moseley GL, Butler DS. Fifteen years of explaining pain: the past, present, and future. J Pain. 2015;16(9):807–13.
34. Louw A, Zimney K, Puentedura EJ, Diener I. The efficacy of pain neuroscience education on musculoskeletal pain: a systematic review of the literature. Physiother Theory Pract. 2016;32(5):332–55.

35. Vibe Fersum K, O'Sullivan P, Skouen J, Smith A, Kvale A. Efficacy of classification based cognitive functional therapy in patients with non specific chronic low back pain: a randomized controlled trial. Eur J Pain. 2013;17(6):916–28.
36. Wilkinson P, Whiteman R. Pain management programmes. BJA CEPD Rev. 2016;17(1):10–5.
37. Durham J, Al-Baghdadi M, Baad-Hansen L, Breckons M, Goulet JP, Lobbezoo F, et al. Self-management programmes in temporomandibular disorders: results from an international Delphi process. J Oral Rehabil. 2016;43(12):929–36.

Psychological Interventions for Persistent Orofacial Pain

5

Sarah Barker, Monika Urbanek, and Chris Penlington

Learning Objectives

- To understand the psychological interventions that can be applied to persistent orofacial pain.
- To consider how these approaches can be applied using a stepped-care model.

Persistent orofacial pain (POFP) is relatively common and affects approximately 10% of adults and up to 50% of the elderly [1]. POFP includes a range of conditions including temporomandibular disorders, burning mouth syndrome, persistent dentoalveolar pain, trigeminal neuralgia, and atypical facial pain [2, 3]. Iatrogenic trigeminal nerve injury can also lead to persistent orofacial pain [4].

Due to the complex anatomy of the region and the difficulties in diagnosis and treatment of chronic pain conditions, the pain is often experienced as recurrent, persistent and disabling [5]. It often presents alongside pain in other body areas [6], suggesting a common pathway with other persistent pain conditions, although there is also some evidence of unique pain pathways in the orofacial region [7].

POFP symptoms have a significant impact on individuals, families and communities. They are often associated with social isolation, psychological distress, sleep disorders, impairment of daily activities, occupational disability, higher frequency of health care use and reduced quality of life [5, 8, 9]. Many patients attending a dental consultation also have co-morbid psychological health issues,

S. Barker (✉) · M. Urbanek
Private Practice, London, UK
e-mail: monikaurbanek@nhs.net

C. Penlington
School of Dental Sciences, Newcastle University, Newcastle upon Tyne, UK
e-mail: Chris.Penlington@newcastle.ac.uk

© The Author(s), under exclusive license to Springer Nature Switzerland AG 2022
T. Renton (ed.), *Optimal Pain Management for the Dental Team*, BDJ Clinician's Guides, https://doi.org/10.1007/978-3-030-86634-1_5

some in the context of other long-term physical health conditions [10]. Identifying and treating these issues can improve dental care, and in the longer term be more financially prudent. Pain is multifactorial, and psychological factors need to be addressed alongside pathology in the dental clinic. The bidirectional relationship between mental and physical health has been hailed as a "new frontier" in healthcare [11] and integrating mental and physical healthcare is now a key priority for clinical commissioning groups (CCGs). Clinical psychologists are increasingly developing a specialised role within dental services, usually working within a multidisciplinary team and carrying out assessments and bespoke interventions for patients with more complex presentations. Interventions led by a clinical psychologist will be shaped and guided by formulation, a key unique skill of clinical psychologists.

5.1   Formulation

Regardless of therapeutic orientation, clinical psychologists are trained to plan and evaluate each intervention based upon an individual formulation for each patient. A formulation is a hypothesis about why a person is experiencing particular problems at a particular time. Thus a formulation is specific to each patient and links theory with practice. It will aim to explain, on the basis of psychological theory, why the particular difficulties experienced by a patient have developed and how they are maintained. In the case of persistent pain, this may refer more to the way in which a patient responds to their pain rather than to the pain itself. It is constructed collaboratively with patients and teams, and guides subsequent interventions, which are based on the psychological processes and principles previously identified. These can subsequently be revised and reformulated.

The roots of the formulation can be traced back to the 1950s when the scientist-practitioner model emerged. The British Psychological Society, in their guidelines on formulation [12] advocates formulating from a broad-based, integrated and multi-model perspective. Recognising wider systemic, organisational and societal influences is key. The process involves reflection and is "a balanced synthesis of the intuitive and rational cognitive systems" [13].

Formulations are seen in terms of their usefulness rather than being a truth [14]. Co-creating a plausible narrative is an ongoing process, and revisions are integral to their application. Corrie and Lane [15] suggested that formulation can also serve other purposes, such as noticing gaps in information, minimising decision-making biases, thinking about lack of progress, helping the person feel understood and contained, and normalising problems.

Formulating is a core competency for clinical psychologists and integral to the way they work. However, this approach can create tensions for research since treatment based on individual formulations by definition cannot be standardised in manuals or fully evaluated by randomised controlled trials.

5.2   Psychological Interventions for Pain

Psychological approaches to persistent pain, described below, include cognitive behaviour therapy (CBT), acceptance and commitment therapy (ACT) and mindfulness-based interventions (MBIs).

Given the increasing demand for psychological care, a stepped care approach is recommended by The National Institute for Health and Care Excellence (NICE). This advocates assessing complexity and tailoring treatment according to need and the resources available. Stepped care for anxiety and depression often involves guided self-help at the lowest intensity, computerised packages of standardised care, group work and individual work of varying duration. We discuss three common psychological approaches below, then outline how these can be implemented within services using a stepped care approach.

5.3   Cognitive Behavioural Therapy

Cognitive behavioural therapy (CBT) for pain management aims to reduce psychological distress and improve physical and role function by helping individuals decrease unhelpful behaviours, increase helpful behaviours, identify and change unhelpful thought patterns and increase self-efficacy for managing pain [16]. For instance, negative thoughts about pain can contribute to the avoidance of pleasant activities and therefore add to emotional distress. The goal of the treatment is to achieve functional recovery outcomes involving improved physical, social and work activity, mood stability, anxiety and sleep disorders [17–19].

It is a present-focused, action-oriented and time-limited intervention. Whilst there are no standard CBT protocols, some of the techniques include relaxation training, setting and working towards behavioural goals, e.g. systematic increases in exercise; behavioural activation, guidance in activity pacing, problem-solving training and cognitive restructuring [20, 21]. Patients are often encouraged to complete activities in between sessions in order to practise new skills, e.g. complete thought records, practise relaxation or work towards behavioural goals [16].

A vast body of research has shown that CBT is effective for a range of chronic pain conditions, including arthritis, sickle cell disease and fibromyalgia. There is also some evidence suggesting benefits for patients with orofacial pain, including temporomandibular dysfunction [22–24]. Turner and colleagues [25] found greater improvements in pain-related beliefs, catastrophising and coping in patients receiving CBT in comparison to a control group. Research has also shown that patients with burning mouth syndrome experience improvements in relation to the severity of pain and discomfort after 12–16 sessions of CBT, and these effects are maintained 6–12 months after therapy [26, 27]. while initial results are promising, further research is required to establish the efficacy of CBT for the orofacial pain conditions.

5.4   Acceptance and Commitment Therapy (ACT)

Acceptance and commitment therapy (ACT) is one of the recent third-wave mindfulness-based behaviour therapies. It was developed in 1982 by Steven C. Hayes who has extensively researched the model and the active processes [28]. It challenges the ground rules of traditional therapeutic approaches, in that it starts from the premise that the psychological processes of a normal human mind are often destructive and can create suffering [29].

ACT is a non-linear model aiming to increase psychological flexibility to effect change [30]. At the centre of an ACT intervention is the "hexaflex", which proposes six processes to achieve psychological flexibility: contact with the present moment, acceptance, values, committed action, self-as-context and defusion. Key questions in this therapy are "what valued direction does the client want to go in" and "what is getting in the way?" in the therapy we continually return to the explicit values the client has and the specific behavioural change they are trying to achieve, whilst building commitment and ensuring the client feels safe. Mindfulness exercises in session can help to build safety. It differs markedly from therapies such as CBT, in that the client is encouraged to defuse thoughts rather than engage with them through evaluation. Metaphors such as "a passing storm" are used to illustrate the impermanence of thoughts and feelings. The ACT model is a shift in focus away from coping methods that emphasise the control or change of psychological experiences, towards acceptance of difficult thoughts and feelings.

ACT is based on functional contextualism, which means we are primarily interested in the function of a particular behaviour. This contrasts with elemental realism on which therapies such as CBT are based, which looks at the form of the behaviour, e.g. whether a particular thought is positive or negative.

Different behaviours can serve the same function, for example, they help the client to avoid painful thoughts and feelings. An ABC approach (antecedents, behaviours and consequences) is a structured way to help bring a mindful approach towards the internal and external antecedents that precede behaviours. Some clients have little self-awareness of their thoughts and feelings before a particular behaviour, and an important part of therapy is to help clients to develop this self-awareness. Helping clients to make links between how they feel, what they do and what is happening physiologically and cognitively can be a key part of therapy. There can be payoffs to destructive behaviours, and these may have provided benefits in the past, but can interfere now and prevent the client from building a rich and meaningful life. Cognitive defusion is used to help clients to gain distance from thoughts and to put painful memories into a historical narrative. There is a range of cognitive defusion techniques, which all aim to create some distance from thoughts. Clients are also encouraged to make "towards" moves to head in the direction of their key values, rather than "away moves". A key aim is to help clients to build their capacity to be in the present moment with openness, curiosity, and flexibility.

An increasing body of literature is demonstrating the effectiveness of this approach in mental health [31] and chronic pain [32]. There is also some evidence that ACT is efficient from a societal or a third-party payer perspective [33]. A recent meta-analysis however noted the low quality of many studies, and the need for high-quality randomised controlled trials (RCTs) [34].

5.5 Mindfulness

Mindfulness-based interventions aim to help people to change their relationship to internal events such as thoughts, feelings and sensations by noticing and accepting present moment experiences without judging or attempting to control them [35]. Mindfulness is considered to be a third-wave approach because the focus for change is not on internal experiences such as thoughts themselves, but on how we relate to these experiences. Mindfulness is a form of meditation that does not aim to promote change or to solve a problem but to develop the capacity to notice present moment experience including thoughts and feelings. This capacity is developed through the regular daily practice of mindfulness meditation. It can help us to develop an awareness of our habitual responses which otherwise tend to be automatic and unseen. As awareness develops, habitual, automatically-driven responses to triggers such as pain or distress reduce and the possibility of actively choosing how to respond helpfully is opened up.

Mindfulness has been extensively used in pain management settings since the pioneering work of Jon Kabat-Zinn who developed mindfulness-based stress reduction (MBSR) [36]. A recent review [37] reported that mindfulness-based interventions showed slight improvements over active or passive control groups in reducing pain intensity and were superior to control groups in reducing depression. No evidence was reported of any difference in efficacy in improving pain or depression between MBIs and other well-established treatments such as CBT. Compassion-focused interventions have been less well studied but also show early promise in pain management settings [38, 39].

5.6 A Stepped Care Approach

Formal psychological measures routinely administered in the clinical setting can offer an indication of levels of anxiety, depression and risk. These measures complement the clinical judgment of therapists involved in patients' care and need to be interpreted in the context of how individuals present in assessment and/or treatment but can be a useful way of stratifying patients for psychological treatment.

Often, people with milder or less entrenched symptoms are considered to be appropriate for structured or manualised therapies using the approaches described, while those with more complex presentations are likely to be referred to clinical psychologists who may be able to address individual blocks to improve with their ability to formulate from a range of therapeutic backgrounds.

Currently, there is seldom a distinction made between higher and lower levels of complexity in research on psychosocial approaches to pain management in POFR it would be useful for this to be reported explicitly in future research since initial complexity is an important variable that affects the outcome. In clinical practice, patients are presenting with increasingly complex presentations, which necessitates close liaison between multidisciplinary colleagues where possible.

Multidisciplinary pain management programmes (PMPs) include psychological input alongside a more physical rehabilitative approach delivered by staff from other disciplines such as physiotherapy, doctors, specialist nurses and occupational therapists. They aim to help patients with more complex presentations of pain which may not have responded to previous treatment.

The psychological components of a PMP are based on CBT or ACT and are delivered alongside other topics including exercise, understanding pain and medication management. A recent Cochrane review [40] reported evidence that PMPs are more effective than usual care (moderate-quality evidence) and physical therapy (low-quality evidence) in terms of pain and disability outcomes that are maintained for at least 12 months post-treatment. There is no evidence to suggest that PMPs are more or less effective than psychological therapies. As discussed, the typically higher level of complexity of patients referred to multidisciplinary treatment would make direct comparisons between the different approaches difficult.

Multidisciplinary programmes developed alongside a recognition that, since pain is multifactorial, no one professional group has the skills to provide successful treatment. Therefore professionals trained in their own discipline have worked together to jointly understand the unique presentations of patients with persistent pain, often adapting methods developed for different contexts for application within a pain management setting. There are exciting developments including neuroscience education (NE) and cognitive functional therapy (CFT), which focus more explicitly on linking an understanding of psychological, biological and contextual factors within a unique formulation for each patient. Claims that the successful application of these biopsychosocial approaches can indeed lead to at least a degree of pain reduction are supported by a review of pain neuroscience education [41] and a randomised controlled trial of CFT [42]. These initially impressive results suggest that both approaches warrant further study and application within POFR.

5.7   Summary

Psychological and multidisciplinary approaches to the management of pain are widely accepted and based on an established scientific rationale. Current evidence consistently describes significant but small improvements in a range of clinical outcomes including pain, disability and depression. Within a stepped care model, the routine administration of psychological measures can aid decisions about which level of treatment is the best fit for a particular patient. This can help to differentiate between people who are suitable for more straightforward, manualised treatment packages and those who require more bespoke interventions due to a higher level of complexity. Within the clinical setting, good quality information and education about the multifactorial nature of pain is essential to ensure that patients appreciate how biological, psychological and social factors impact on each other.

References

1. Madland G, Newton-John T, Feinmann C. Facial pain: chronic idiopathic orofacial pain: I: What is the evidence base? Br Dent J. 2001;191(1):22.
2. Macfarlane T, Glenny A, Worthington H. Systematic review of population-based epidemiological studies of oro-facial pain. J Dent. 2001;29(7):451–67.
3. de Leeuw R, Klasser GD. Orofacial pain: guidelines for assessment, diagnosis, and management. Chicago: Quintessence; 2008.
4. Hillerup S. Iatrogenic injury to oral branches of the trigeminal nerve: records of 449 cases. Clin Oral Investig. 2007;11(2):133–42.
5. Oberoi SS, Hiremath S, Yashoda R, Marya C, Rekhi A. Prevalence of various orofacial pain symptoms and their overall impact on quality of life in a Tertiary Care Hospital in India. J Maxillofacial Oral Surg. 2014;13(4):533–8.
6. Maixner W, Diatchenko L, Dubner R, Fillingim RB, Greenspan JD, Knott C, et al. Orofacial pain prospective evaluation and risk assessment study-the OPPERA study. J Pain. 2011;12(11):T4–T11.e2.
7. Rodriguez E, Sakurai K, Xu J, Chen Y, Toda K, Zhao S, et al. A craniofacial-specific monosynaptic circuit enables heightened affective pain. Nat Neurosci. 2017;20(12):1734–43.
8. Wan K, McMillan A, Wong M. Orofacial pain symptoms and associated disability and psychosocial impact in community-dwelling and institutionalized elderly in Hong Kong. Community Dent Health. 2012;29(1):110–6.
9. Shueb S, Nixdorf D, John M, Alonso BF, Durham J. What is the impact of acute and chronic orofacial pain on quality of life? J Dent. 2015;43(10):1203–10.
10. Naylor C, Parsonage M, McDaid D, Knapp M, Fossey M, Galea A. Long term conditions and mental health; the cost of co-morbidities. London: The Kings Fund Centre for Mental Health; 2012.
11. Naylor C, Das P, Ross S, Honeyman M, Thompson J, Gilburt H. Bringing together physical and mental health. London: The Kings Fund Centre for Mental Health; 2018.
12. The British Psychological Society. Good practice guidelines on the use of psychological formulation. Leicester, UK: British Psychological Society; 2011.
13. Kuyken W. Evidence-based case formulation: is the emperor clothed? Case formulation in cognitive behaviour therapy. London: Routledge; 2006. p. 28–51.
14. Johnstone L. Controversies and debates about formulation. Formulation in psychology and psychotherapy. London: Routledge; 2006. p. 225–52.
15. Corrie S. Constructing stories, telling tales: a guide to formulation in applied psychology. London: Routledge; 2018.
16. Ehde DM, Dillworth TM, Turner JA. Cognitive-behavioral therapy for individuals with chronic pain: efficacy, innovations, and directions for research. Am Psychol. 2014;69(2):153.
17. Alsaadi SM, McAuley JH, Hush JM, Maher CG. Prevalence of sleep disturbance in patients with low back pain. Eur Spine J. 2011;20(5):737–43.
18. Coupland M. CBT for pain management. Int Assoc Ind Accid Boards Comm (IAIABC). 2009;6(2):77–91.
19. Gore M, Sadosky A, Stacey BR, Tai K-S, Leslie D. The burden of chronic low back pain: clinical comorbidities, treatment patterns, and health care costs in usual care settings. Spine. 2012;37(11):E668–E77.
20. Turner JARJM. Cognitive-behavioral therapy for chronic pain. In: Loeser JDBJJ, editor. Bonica's management of pain. 3rd ed. Philadelphia, PA: Lippincott Williams & Wilkins; 2001. p. 1751–8.
21. Thorn BE. Cognitive therapy for chronic pain: a step-by-step guide. New York: Guilford Publications; 2017.
22. Kotiranta U, Suvinen T, Forssell H. Tailored treatments in temporomandibular disorders: where are we now? A systematic qualitative literature review. J Oral Facial Pain Headache. 2014;28(1):28–37.

23. Randhawa K, Bohay R, Côté P, van der Velde G, Sutton D, Wong JJ, et al. The effectiveness of noninvasive interventions for temporomandibular disorders. Clin J Pain. 2016;32(3):260–78.
24. List T, Axelsson S. Management of TMD: evidence from systematic reviews and meta-analyses. J Oral Rehabil. 2010;37(6):430–51.
25. Turner JA, Mancl L, Aaron LA. Brief cognitive-behavioral therapy for temporomandibular disorder pain: effects on daily electronic outcome and process measures. Pain. 2005;117(3):377–87.
26. Bergdahl J, Anneroth G, Ferris H. Cognitive therapy in the treatment of patients with resistant burning mouth syndrome: a controlled study. J Oral Pathol Med. 1995;24(5):213–5.
27. Femiano F, Gombos F, Scully C. Burning mouth syndrome: open trial of psychotherapy alone, medication with alpha-lipoic acid (thioctic acid), and combination therapy. Medicina Oral. 2004;9(1):8–13.
28. Hayes SC, Luoma JB, Bond FW, Masuda A, Lillis J. Acceptance and commitment therapy: model, processes and outcomes. Behav Res Ther. 2006;44(1):1–25.
29. Harris R. The happiness trap: stop struggling, start living. London: Exisle Publishing; 2013.
30. Trompetter HR, Bohlmeijer ET, Fox J-P, Schreurs KM. Psychological flexibility and catastrophizing as associated change mechanisms during online Acceptance & Commitment Therapy for chronic pain. Behav Res Ther. 2015;74:50–9.
31. A-tjak JG, Davis ML, Morina N, Powers MB, Smits JA, Emmelkamp PM. A meta-analysis of the efficacy of acceptance and commitment therapy for clinically relevant mental and physical health problems. Psychother Psychosom. 2015;84(1):30–6.
32. Simpson PA, Mars T, Esteves JE. A systematic review of randomised controlled trials using Acceptance and commitment therapy as an intervention in the management of non-malignant, chronic pain in adults. Int J Osteopathic Med. 2017;24:18–31.
33. Feliu-Soler A, Cebolla A, McCracken LM, D'Amico F, Knapp M, Lopez-Montoyo A, et al. Economic impact of third-wave cognitive behavioral therapies: a systematic review and quality assessment of economic evaluations in randomized controlled trials. Behav Ther. 2018;49(1):124–47.
34. Graham CD, Gouick J, Krahe C, Gillanders D. A systematic review of the use of Acceptance and Commitment Therapy (ACT) in chronic disease and long-term conditions. Clin Psychol Rev. 2016;46:46–58.
35. Kabat Zinn J. Some reflections on the origins of MBSR, skillful means, and the trouble with maps. Contemp Buddhism. 2011;12(1):281–306.
36. Kabat-Zinn J, Lipworth L, Burney R, Sellers W, Brew M. Reproducibility and four year follow-up of a training program in mindfulness meditation for the self-regulation of chronic pain. Pain. 1984;18:S303.
37. Hilton L, Hempel S, Ewing BA, Apaydin E, Xenakis L, Newberry S, et al. Mindfulness meditation for chronic pain: systematic review and meta-analysis. Ann Behav Med. 2017;51(2):199–213.
38. Chapin HL, Darnall BD, Seppala EM, Doty JR, Hah JM, Mackey SC. Pilot study of a compassion meditation intervention in chronic pain. J Compassionate Health Care. 2014;1(1):1.
39. Penlington C. Exploring a compassion-focused intervention for persistent pain in a group setting. Br J Pain. 2018;2018:2049463718772148.
40. Kamper SJ, Apeldoorn A, Chiarotto A, Smeets R, Ostelo R, Guzman J, et al. Multidisciplinary biopsychosocial rehabilitation for chronic low back pain: Cochrane systematic review and metaanalysis. BMJ. 2015;350:h444.
41. Louw A, Zimney K, Puentedura EJ, Diener I. The efficacy of pain neuroscience education on musculoskeletal pain: a systematic review of the literature. Physiother Theory Pract. 2016;32(5):332–55.
42. Vibe Fersum K, O'Sullivan P, Skouen J, Smith A, Kvale A. Efficacy of classification based cognitive functional therapy in patients with non specific chronic low back pain: a randomized controlled trial. Eur J Pain. 2013;17(6):916–28.

An Overview of Dental Anxiety and the Non-pharmacological Management of Dental Anxiety

6

Jennifer Hare, Geanina Bruj-Milasan, and Tim Newton

Learning Objectives

- An overview of the definition, prevalence and management of dental anxiety and phobia, and knowledge of:
  - The definition of dental anxiety, and the diagnostic features of dental phobia.
  - The prevalence of mild, moderate and severe dental anxiety.
  - Managing anxiety in dental settings.

Anxiety has been defined as a "vague, unpleasant feeling accompanied by a premonition that something undesirable is about to happen" [1]. Although the terms "anxiety" and "fear" are often used interchangeably, anxiety is usually said to be a general feeling whereas fear is termed a reaction to a specific event or object. In reality, this can be a difficult distinction to draw and many authors use the two terms interchangeably. However, for the purposes of this article, we will tend to use the term "dental anxiety" to refer to mild and moderate negative feelings about dentistry, including the dental environment and dental treatment, and dental phobia as the most severe form of such fear.

The level of anxiety an individual experiences in relation to dental treatment is likely to vary from person to person. Some will experience low levels of anxiety, while others more moderate levels up to and including those with phobic levels of anxiety. The term "phobia" is reserved for an anxiety disorder comprising a marked and specific fear that is excessive or unreasonable. The DSM-V [2] criteria for the diagnosis of dental phobia are:

- Considerable and persistent fear in response to the presence or anticipation of a specific object or situation (in this instance the dental setting or dental treatment).

J. Hare (✉) · G. Bruj-Milasan · T. Newton
Dental Psychology Service, Guy's and St Thomas NHS Foundation Trust, London, UK
e-mail: Jennifer.Hare@gstt.nhs.uk; geanina.bruj@gstt.nhs.uk; tim.newton@kcl.ac.uk

© The Author(s), under exclusive license to Springer Nature Switzerland AG 2022
T. Renton (ed.), *Optimal Pain Management for the Dental Team*, BDJ Clinician's
Guides, https://doi.org/10.1007/978-3-030-86634-1_6

- Exposure to the stimulus almost always evokes an instant anxiety response.
- The individual recognises that the fear is unreasonable or excessive.
- The phobic object/situation is either avoided or endured with strong anxiety.
- The fear, anticipatory anxiety or avoidance behaviour interferes with social or occupational functioning or daily routines **or** there is considerable distress about having this phobia.
- The phobia must be of a duration greater than 6 months.
- The symptoms cannot be better explained by any other diagnosis.

The ICD-10 [3] criteria for dental phobia are similar but simpler:

- The symptoms represent primary manifestations of anxiety rather than being symptoms of obsessional or delusional thoughts.
- The anxiety is circumscribed to a particular object or situation.
- The feared object or situation is avoided where possible.

The Five Areas™ model of anxiety suggests that anxiety has five elements comprising: situational factors, unhelpful thoughts, unhelpful behaviours, physical symptoms and feelings [4]. The dental setting is a complex situation that may have many triggers to anxiety including the sounds and smells associated with the dental surgery, as well as specific aspects of dental treatment. For example, fear of injections is one of the most common aspects of dental phobia [5]. Furthermore the level of dental anxiety demonstrated by a patient is likely to be an interaction of their general feelings about dentistry, and the specific dental challenge they are facing at that time.

The physiological manifestations of anxiety are typically mediated through the autonomic nervous system—increased heart rate, sweating, raised blood pressure, palpitations and breathlessness. Perhaps the most common behavioural manifestation of anxiety is avoidance of the anxiety-provoking situation or escape from the situation, and this is recognised in the definitions of the phobia within the DSM and ICD classifications. There are other behavioural manifestations, including some patients who report attempts at meticulous oral hygiene in order to maintain oral health and therefore lessen the need for visiting a dentist [6], or disruptive behaviour during the dental visit. Cognitive elements of anxiety include both unhelpful thoughts about the situation (e.g. what could go wrong) and also the impact of anxiety on our thinking processes. For instance, anxiety may reduce our ability to concentrate or to remember.

6.1   The Prevalence of Dental Anxiety and Phobia

The prevalence of phobic levels of anxiety appears to be consistently in the region of 10% of the population, though the prevalence of dental phobia is higher in women than men, but tends to decline in prevalence after the age of 50. A review of the published epidemiological studies of dental anxiety and phobia in adults is provided by Raadal and Skarat [7].

The prevalence of low and moderate levels of dental anxiety is more difficult to determine. Hill et al. [5] defined low, moderate and severe anxiety using cut-offs for the modified dental anxiety scale (MDAS) in a sample of 10,900 UK adults. Low levels of anxiety were reported in 51% of adults, 36% had an MDAS score of between 10 and 18 indicating moderate dental anxiety, and a further 12% had a score of 19 or more which suggests extreme dental anxiety.

6.2   Comorbidity in Dental Anxiety

Individuals with dental phobia often experience a range of other psychological problems in addition to their extreme anxiety. General anxiety is common—occurring in approximately 40% of patients with dental phobia [8], depression has been also reported—though at levels which might be expected in the general population. Other commonly found comorbidities include the presence of blood-injury-injection phobia (BII) where the individual has a marked reaction to injury, the sight of blood, or injections of any form. Often in the instance of BII, the fear of dental treatment may be simply a manifestation of a fear that dental treatment may involve one or more of these elements. Post-traumatic stress disorder has been reported in some individuals who have the clear manifestation of PTSD in relation to dental settings, for example, flashbacks. Kani et al. [8] also report that approximately 3% of their patient group reported suicidal ideation in the last month prior to their assessment for dental phobia.

6.3   The Impact of Dental Phobia

Living with an extreme fear of dental treatment appears to have a broad range of impacts on the individual, from the predictable impact on the oral health of prolonged avoidance of dental treatment to the less apparent impacts on social and psychological wellbeing.

6.3.1   Oral Health

Individuals with dental phobia have poorer oral health than those who are not dentally phobic. A review of epidemiological studies of non-clinical populations found that in general there is a clear gradient in the relationship between the level of dental anxiety and oral health, with increased anxiety at all levels being associated with poorer oral health [9], across all measures including self-reported oral health, oral health-related quality of life, caries rates, tooth loss and periodontal disease. Individuals with dental phobia presenting for treatment at specialist centres have been found to have markedly poorer oral health, a finding likely to be due to the observation that the patients' eventual presentation for treatment is triggered by their deteriorating condition [10, 11].

6.3.2   Psychosocial Functioning

Though less extensively researched, there is some evidence that people with dental phobia may experience some impact on their daily functioning and quality of life. Cohen et al. [6] undertook a series of qualitative interviews with individuals attending a specialist treatment centre for individuals with dental phobia and reported a number of impacts among this group. Similarly, epidemiological surveys reveal elevated levels of embarrassment, impaired social functioning (smiling in social situations, etc.) and impaired quality of life amongst individuals with extreme dental fear [12–14]. Increased medication use, low self-confidence and self-esteem, psychosomatic disorders and increased time off work have also been reported amongst people with dental phobia compared to non-dentally phobic populations [11]. Hägglin et al. [15] reported that women with high levels of dental anxiety reported significantly impaired social functioning on the SF-36 in comparison to non-phobic women, notably in the areas of physical function, pain perceived general health, vitality, social functions, mental health and emotional well-being.

6.4   Impact on the Dental Team

Dealing with patients who are anxious about dental treatment has been reported as a source of stress for the dental team [16]. This impact may occur both through the additional time requirements in order to implement care and coping strategies for an individual who is anxious, as well as the interpersonal stress of working with someone who is in distress. The additional time required for managing an individual with high levels of anxiety may lead to running late with subsequent patients and the difficulties that follow. It is acknowledged that having to reassure a patient who may have very negative perceptions of your role is in itself stressful [16].

6.5   The Proportionate Model of Anxiety Management

Newton et al. [17] outline a stepped approach to intervention for people with dental anxiety which intensifies the level of intervention according to the level of anxiety reported by the patient (Fig. 6.1).

   We believe that these approaches can be grouped into combinations for applicability in the dental setting, as follows:

6.5.1   Adopt a Preventive and Minimally Invasive Approach
         to Caries Management

Given that many people who are dentally anxious report having traumatic experiences (e.g. considerable pain, invasive treatment, humiliation, loss of control) at the dentist earlier in their life [18–20], it can be hypothesised that a more preventive

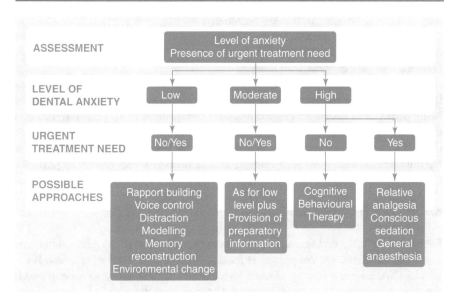

Fig. 6.1 The proportionate model of dental anxiety

approach associated with less invasive treatment (such as interim restorative care) should also have a positive influence on anxiety about dental visits. This approach is as yet untested but is aligned with developments in minimally invasive dentistry [21].

6.5.2   Create a Warm and Welcoming Environment Conducive to Cooperation

The environment of dental surgery has been identified as a barrier for patients accessing dental services, in particular patients' perceptions of the attitudes and values of the staff. Fundamental to this would be staff training in communication skills so that each patient is welcomed in a warm and sympathetic way, creating a seamless journey from the reception to the dental surgery. In addition, consider the images and smells of the practice and how these may help to calm the patient [17].

6.5.3   Build Rapport and Trust

The primary technique that we recommend to build rapport and trust in adult patients is the use of structured formats to start a discussion on how the dental team and patient can work together to identify what steps can be taken to make the patient feel more comfortable during their dental treatment. Clinically we work with patients to write a "letter to the dentist" in which they outline techniques, which they feel could be helpful to them personally, for example: being able to listen to music, taking regular breaks, the use of an agreed stop signal, etc. Obviously, the clinical team and the patient need to agree on what is feasible and realistic. Both clinician and patient agree with the list.

For adolescents and young adults, recent research has successfully demonstrated the power of using pro forma communication tools to enhance children's sense of being involved in decisions concerning their care. Porritt et al. [22] designed and tested an intervention designed to enable young people aged 10–16 to work with their dentist to devise a care plan for their anxiety. The benefits that accrued from the intervention were both immediate and maintained at 1-year follow-up [23].

6.5.4 Teach Coping Skills

Feelings of anxiety and fear are made worse by a number of thoughts and beliefs about the situation that the person is facing; for example, anxiety is worse if the person affected has a feeling of uncertainty about what is going to happen and if the person feels that they have little or no control over the situation. Anxiety also results in a shift in thought processes to an increased awareness of sights, sounds and sensations (hypervigilance), as well as a tendency to focus on the negative aspects of the dental situation. The techniques outlined below share the common approach of teaching the individual techniques to cope with their anxiety through learning more about what is going to happen, sharing the control over the situation with their clinician, decreasing vigilance and attending to the more positive aspects of dental care.

Attention shifting or distraction: Several types of distraction have been reported in the literature, including the use of video-taped cartoons, audio-taped stories and video games. Distraction techniques have been found to be as effective as relaxation-based techniques, and superior to no intervention. Recent advances in technology have also seen encouraging results with the use of virtual reality (VR) head-mounted display devices (HMD) used for distraction, which have demonstrated encouraging reductions in anxiety and pain perceptions among children shown videos on virtual glasses [24] and among adults immersed in virtual environments [25].

Uncertainty is anxiety-provoking, and can be reduced by providing preparatory information and by enhancing an individual's sense of control over the situation. One widely used technique to do this is the "stop" signal which has been shown to be effective in dental settings and a wide variety of other medical settings [26]. The clinician and patient agree on a sign (usually the raising of a hand), which signals that the patient wishes the clinician to stop treatment for a period of time.

Providing information on what is likely to happen during a dental visit is a useful way of decreasing the uncertainty around the visit. Such information could be provided to the parent or carer to share in an age-appropriate manner. Methods of delivering preparatory information might include written information, books or short videos. A systematic review of the effectiveness of preparatory information [27] suggests that information on three aspects of the treatment are important:

- What will happen (procedural)
- What sensations the individual will experience (sensory)
- What the individual can do to cope with the situation (coping).

An example might be the giving of a local anaesthetic injection. Information can be given about the sensations the individual will experience—for example although there is no sensation in the injected area, the patient will still be able to feel vibration and pressure. Typically this takes 2–5 min to start and lasts up to 2 h. When the injection fades, the sensation is similar to "pins and needles" which the patient will have experienced. Video may provide an excellent way to provide such preparatory information, provided it follows the guidelines above and is approved by the clinician as accurate and reflecting their own practice.

6.5.5 Reward Effort

Acknowledging the patient's achievement in making progress towards dental treatment in the face of their anxiety is an important way to reward the effort that they have made. Patients should be praised for specific behaviours that build towards achieving their goals in terms of dental anxiety: for example rather than praising a patient for "doing well", the clinician should praise them for "completing the examination". In general, for children, tangible rewards are more effective than intangible rewards though praise and attention should also be used together with tangible rewards. Research from our team [28] suggests that if given the choice of a reward, children tend to choose tangible rewards, and that parents are poor at predicting what rewards children might use. The use of rewards is appropriate across all age ranges, though the type of reward will vary.

6.6 Refer for Guidance of Severe Levels of Dental Phobia and Behaviour Guidance Problems

The use of Cognitive Behavioural Therapy for Dental Phobia has been shown to be highly effective in enabling patients to attend dental treatment in the long term without pharmacological interventions such as sedation or general anaesthesia [29]. Whilst pharmacological interventions enable urgent dental treatment to be undertaken comfortably, they are only minimally effective in helping the individual to overcome their dental fear. CBT provides a framework for rehabilitating the individual's dental fear and enabling them to attend dental treatment without sedation or general anaesthetic. Provision of CT for dental phobia is a specialised service, the details of which are beyond the scope of this article [29].

6.7 Summary

Dental anxiety is a common and dental phobia, the most extreme form of dental fear, affects approximately 10% of the population. A further 36% of the population are moderately anxious about visiting the dentist and receiving dental practice. Furthermore, the degree of invasiveness of the dental treatment may lead to further anxiety. The impact of dental anxiety and phobia is marked, affecting health and wellbeing. The management of patients who are concerned about dental treatment should follow these principles: adopt a preventive and minimally invasive approach to caries management; create a warm and welcoming environment conducive to cooperation; build rapport and trust; teach coping skills; reward effort; refer for the guidance of severe levels of dental phobia and behaviour guidance problems.

References

1. Kagan J, Havemann E. Psychology. An introduction. New York: Harcourt Brace Jovanavich; 1976.
2. American Psychiatric Association. Diagnostic and statistical manual of mental disorders. 5th ed, text revision. Washington DC: American Psychiatric Association; 2002.
3. World Health Organisation. The ICD-10 classification of mental and behavioural disorders. Clinical descriptions and diagnostic guidelines. Geneva: World Health Organisation; 1992.
4. Williams C, Garland A. A cognitive-behavioural therapy assessment model for use in everyday clinical practice. Adv Psychiatr Treat. 2002;8:172–9.
5. Hill KB. Dental anxiety and the oral health of the population. Social Sci Dent. 2012;3:10–4.
6. Cohen SM, Fiske J, Newton JT. The impact of dental anxiety on daily living. Br Dent J. 2000;189(7):385–90.
7. Raadal M, Skarat E. Background description and epidemiology. In: Öst L-G, Skarat E, editors. Cognitive behavior therapy for dental phobia and anxiety. Chichester: John Wiley & Sons Ltd; 2013. p. 21–32.
8. Kani E, Asimakopoulou K, Daly B, Hare J, Lewis J, Scambler S, Scott S, Newton JT. Characteristics of patients attending for Cognitive Behavioural Therapy at one specialist unit for dental phobia in the UK and outcomes of treatment. Br Dent J. 2015;219:501–6.
9. Hakeberg M, Lundgren J. Symptoms, clinical characteristics and consequences. In: Öst L-G, Skarat E, editors. Cognitive behavior therapy for dental phobia and anxiety. Chichester: John Wiley & Sons Ltd; 2013. p. 3–20.
10. Agdal ML, Raadal M, Skarat E, Kvale G. Oral health and oral treatment needs in patients fulfilling the DSM-IV criteria for dental phobia: possible influence on the outcome of cognitive behavioural therapy. Acta Odontol Scand. 2008;66:1–6.
11. Wide Boman U, Lundgren J, Berggren U, Carlsson SG. Psychosocial and dental factors in the maintenance of severe dental fear. Swed Dent J. 2010;34:121–7.
12. Berggren U. Psychosocial effects associated with dental fear in adult dental populations with avoidance behaviours. Psychol Health. 2003;8:185–96.
13. Locker D. Psychosocial consequences of dental fear and anxiety. Community Dent Oral Epidemiol. 2003;31:144–51.
14. Croft-Barnes NP, Brough E, Wilson KE, Beddis AJ, Girdler NM. Anxiety and quality of life in phobic dental patients. J Dent Res. 2010;89:302–6.
15. Hägglin C, Hakeberg M, Ahlqvist M, Sullivan M, Berggren U. Factors associated with dental anxiety and attendance in middle-aged and elderly women in Sweden. Community Dent Oral Epidemiol. 2000;28:451–60.

16. Newton T, Mistry K, Patel A, Patel P, Perkins M, Saeed K, Smith C. Stress in dental specialists: a comparison of six clinical dental specialities. Prim Dent Care. 2002;9:100–4.
17. Newton JT, Asimakopoulou K, Daly B, Scambler S, Scott S. The management of dental anxiety: time for a sense of proportion? Br Dent J. 2012;213:271–4.
18. Shaw O. Dental anxiety in children. Br Dent J. 1975;139:134–9.
19. Lautch H. Dental phobia. Br J Psychiatry. 1971;119:151–8.
20. Vassend O. Anxiety, pain and discomfort associated with dental treatment. Behav Res Therapy. 1993;31:659–66.
21. Banerjee A. Minimally invasive operative caries management: rationale and techniques. Br Dent J. 2013;214:107–11.
22. Porritt J, Rodd H, Morgan A, Williams C, Gupta E, Kirby J, Cresswell C, Newton JT, Stevens K, Baker S, Prasad S, Marshman Z. Development and testing of a Cognitive Behavioral Therapy resource for children's dental anxiety. JDR Clin Transl Res. 2017;2:23–37.
23. Rodd H, Kirby J, Duffy E, Porritt J, Morgan A, Prasad S, Baker S, Marshman Z. Children's experiences following a CBT intervention to reduce dental anxiety: one year on. Br Dent J. 2018;225:247–51.
24. Aminabadi NA, Erfanparast L, Sohrabi A, Oskouei SG, Naghili A. The impact of virtual reality distraction on pain and anxiety during dental treatment in 4–5 year-old children: a randomised controlled clinical trial. J Dent Res Dent Clin Dent Prospects. 2012;6(4):117–24.
25. Wiederhold MD, Gao K, Widerhold BK. Clinical use of virtual reality distraction system to reduce anxiety and pain in dental procedures. Cyberpsychol Behav Soc Netw. 2014;17(6):359–65.
26. Richardson PH, Black NJ, Justins DM, Watson RJD. The use of stop signals to reduce the pain and distress of patients undergoing a stressful medical procedure: an exploratory clinical study. Br J Med Psychol. 2009;72:397–405.
27. Jaaniste T, Hayes B, von Baeyer CL. Providing children with information about forthcoming medical procedures: a review and synthesis. Clin Psychol Sci Pract. 2007;14:124–43.
28. Coxon J, Hosey MT, Newton JT. What reward does a child prefer for behaving well at the dentist? Br Dent J Open. 2017;3:17018.
29. Newton JT, Gallagher JE. The care and cure of dental phobia: the use of cognitive behaviour therapy to complement conscious sedation. Faculty Dent J. 2018;8:160–3.

Medical Management of Dental Anxiety

7

Paul Coulthard

Learning Objectives

- To describe the current state of sedation practice.
- To discuss the recent publications and guidance in the United Kingdom.
- To describe the responsibility of the clinician in risk assessment and clinical decision-making rather than following prescriptive protocols.

Patients rightly expect that any pain and anxiety associated with their dental care is adequately managed. Undergraduate dental education recognises this expectation and practising clinicians are experienced in managing these aspects of care that are fundamental to the practice of dentistry. Sadly, the prevalence of dental anxiety has not reduced over recent decades and persists in developed societies. A recent telephone survey of 12,000 individuals in England found that 17% did not attend regular dental care and that the main reason for non-attendance was anxiety [1]. Medical management of dental anxiety is therefore important to facilitate access to dental care as well as in supporting high-quality care.

Empathy is an essential characteristic required of any dental practitioner and selection procedures for undergraduate dental and other healthcare programmes now attempt to identify a caring attitude. So is "medical management" of dental anxiety necessary? Patients present with a huge range of issues beyond their particular "dental" needs [2]. Whole patient care is normal and includes identifying not only the relevant general health history but also the individual psychosocial complexities including anxiety for dental care. The patient may volunteer their anxiety or may not. The role of the dental practitioner is to identify all issues, including anxiety, that may be relevant to how oral care is to be delivered and to plan treatment

P. Coulthard (✉)
Institute of Dentistry, Barts and The London School of Medicine and Dentistry, Queen Mary University of London, London, UK
e-mail: p.coulthard@qmul.ac.uk

© The Author(s), under exclusive license to Springer Nature Switzerland AG 2022
T. Renton (ed.), *Optimal Pain Management for the Dental Team*, BDJ Clinician's Guides, https://doi.org/10.1007/978-3-030-86634-1_7

accordingly. The majority of patients need no special adjustment to their treatment delivery and dental team empathy is all that is required. For many patients, "tell, show and do" behavioural management is sufficient and effective in alleviating anxiety. Dentists and their team members become proficient in providing patients with a greater sense of control during treatment if required, as well as distraction, and use of non-threatening language as appropriate.

For some patients, empathy and behavioural management techniques are not sufficient to alleviate their anxiety, and medical or drug management is necessary to avoid distress. For some patients, cognitive behavioural therapy (CBT) may be appropriate. Fortunately, we have drugs available that are effective in reducing dental anxiety and that have demonstrated an excellent safety record over many decades. The definition of UK conscious sedation has not changed for many years and is useful in describing the purpose, patient benefit and safety: "A technique in which the use of a drug or drugs produces a state of depression of the central nervous system enabling treatment to be carried out, but during which verbal contact is maintained throughout the period of sedation. The drugs and techniques used to provide conscious sedation should carry a margin of safety wide enough to render loss of consciousness unlikely. The level of consciousness must be such that the patient remains conscious, retains protective reflexes, and is able to understand and respond to verbal commands" [3].

7.1 Risks and Benefits of Guidance and Regulations

An important duty for the dental practitioner is to make an appropriate assessment to determine whether a patient will be adequately managed for their dental treatment with empathy and behavioural management strategies alone or will require medical management with conscious sedation [4]. A patient experiencing distress will seek care with another dental practitioner or avoid future care completely and develop a phobia, that is, an exaggerated level of anxiety relating to future dental care.

The need for the management of dental anxiety with drugs is not new and numerous techniques have been developed over the past 100 years or more. This area of dental practice has been subject to a disproportionate number of guidelines and regulations. Conscious sedation practice within the NHS has also been significantly influenced by changes to payment systems over the years. Patients have not always been best served as a consequence and access to sedation services via the NHS has been more limited over the past decade.

The publication in 2015 of *Standards for Conscious Sedation in the Provision of Dental Care: Report of the Intercollegiate Advisory Committee for Sedation in Dentistry (IACSD)* [3] provided a much-needed update on clinical practice guidelines, but unfortunately resulted in the unintended consequence of reducing patient access to conscious sedation services, with some dentists abandoning their provision of sedation techniques, believing that they did not satisfy the new training requirements. In fact, the training requirements proposed were only for dentists seeking to start offering sedation techniques and not for those already offering these techniques—but there was considerable misunderstanding and confusion.

A subsequent publication in 2017, *Conscious Sedation in Dentistry—Dental Clinical Guidance* by the Scottish Dental Clinical Effectiveness Programme (SDCEP) referenced the 2015 Standards publication and offered clarity to clinicians around practice [5]. The 2017 publication also emphasised the quality, good and poor, of the research evidence supporting recommended practice. SDCEP used rigorous methodology for the development of recommendations following the GRADE (grading of recommendations, assessment, development and evaluation) approach (www.gradeworkinggroup.org). Key recommendations were developed through considered judgments made by the working group based on previous guidelines but updated as appropriate in the light of the available evidence, whilst taking into account clinical experience, expert opinion and patient and practitioner perspectives. This 2017 guidance went someway to encourage a reversal in the decline in sedation services.

The 2015 *Standards* document offers detailed guidance of the appropriate levels of training required according to the technique and patient age (Sect. 5 and Appendix 1) [3]. Transitional arrangements were described for experienced dentists, sedationists and dental nurses for whom re-training and/or additional qualifications are not necessary. Clinicians are required to maintain a logbook of clinical cases; undertake validated relevant continuing professional development; audit; have skills to manage adverse events; meet the described requirements for the environment and ensure appropriate clinical governance is in place. The training recommendations apply to doctors, dental hygienists, dental therapists and dental nurses in addition to dentists.

For "new starters" in conscious sedation provision, training should be obtained through an accredited provider on a list held by the Sedation Training Accreditation Committee (STAC) of the Faculty of Dental Surgery of the Royal College of Surgeons of England [3].

7.2 Children and Young People

The vast majority of sedation for dental care is offered as nitrous oxide with oxygen by inhalation or with the benzodiazepine, midazolam, administered intravenously. Both techniques titrate the drug dose against the patient response and have been widely and safely used for many years [6]. Other drugs and techniques are also used and may be appropriate in special circumstances. Intranasal midazolam, for example, is used for patients with special needs. This more unusual route of administration has become acceptable because of its demonstrated effectiveness and safety. Increasing commitment to maintaining optimal patient safety on conscious sedation use in dentistry leads to the production of guidance with training recommendations for those using mainstay standard techniques and for those dentists or doctors using "advanced" or "alternative" sedation techniques. The most recent publication in England was published in 2017 and specifically described a "service standard" for conscious sedation in the primary care setting [7]. This had important implications for practice in limiting sedation techniques for patients aged under 16 years. The "service standard" was written to support commissioners of services in England and reflected safety concerns about the use of multi-drug sedation techniques in the young patient population. It stated that for new service procurements multi-drug sedation would no longer be funded in the NHS for patients under 16 years of age.

7.3 Who Needs Medical Management of Anxiety and Who Doesn't?

Traditionally, dental and medical treatment options have been offered to patients according to the clinician's individual knowledge and experience, and any special interest or not, in a particular area of practice. This was the case for conscious sedation in dentistry. There was a wide range of recommended treatment options for care for patients according to the clinician seen. Whilst it is accepted that there is often more than one way to manage a patient's needs, it became clear that some patients were being denied access to conscious sedation services that they needed whilst others were receiving such management that they did not need. In the latter situation, it was thought that sedation services had become "demand-lead" rather than decision-making is based on actual patient "need" [8]. This was the same situation as had been observed in the past with general anaesthesia services in the United Kingdom. The particular concern was, however, that many patients may not have been offered sedation when they needed it because of restrictions as described above in addition to clinician decision-making bias. This might go some way to explaining why the prevalence of dental anxiety had not reduced in England over time.

The author, with others, set about developing a tool to challenge clinician decision-making in the hope of improving the quality of the decision for the patient. The indicator of sedation need (IOSN) tool was developed and first published in 2011 [9]. The tool simply described the well-accepted indications for sedation of a patient's anxiety, medical and behavioural status and treatment complexity, but provided more objectivity with numeric scoring. The "anxiety measure" part of the tool is to be completed by the patient and not the clinician, to add to the objectivity. The IOSN was intended to support and challenge individual clinical decision-making, with particular benefit in the training and education situation.

The NHS in the United Kingdom and other health care systems internationally were starting to expect more objective clinical decision-making, more equitable access to patient services, and greater consideration of cost-effectiveness. The development of the IOSN was timely. In addition to supporting individual patient decision-making, the tool could also be used to look at whole populations. It was found that 5.1% of patients regularly attending general dental practices in England had a high need for conscious sedation. When including those who don't attend regularly, then the likely conscious sedation need was found to be 6.7% of the population [10] This is very helpful for commissioners and service development to provide an idea of the likely requirements. For more invasive treatment than general dental care, such as oral surgery, the need will of course be much higher.

It should be noted that both the IOSN tool and the modified dental anxiety scale that is incorporated, have been tested on adult populations only and is currently only suitable for decision-making in patients aged 16 years or over [11].

7.4   Current Clinical Controversies

The practice of conscious sedation may appear to have changed little as described by the recent relevant publications, but actually, the way in which various issues are to be addressed has changed significantly. Rather than a textbook "cookbook" description detailing the methodology of the technique, the responsibility is for the clinician to risk assess and make informed clinical decisions about sedation methodology. This is a more appropriate way to manage individual patients and tailor the technique. This approach requires clinicians to use their knowledge and experience to determine the best management strategy for a particular patient rather than default to a prescribed protocol. This more flexible approach is new and supports intelligent freedom for clinicians making decisions.

Patients have traditionally not been required by UK dental practitioners to starve from food or fluids prior to dental sedation whilst the same patient would be required to starve as per general anaesthesia if the sedation has been provided by an anaesthetist. This area was therefore seen to be controversial. Current advice is to assess the risk for the individual patient when making a recommendation around this preoperative preparation. Typically, most patients will not be required by their dental practitioner to starve, but there may be an occasion when fasting is appropriate and a generic no-starvation policy is not in the safety interests of every patient. This more flexible and pragmatic approach reflects a new way of practising. In this era of evidence-based practice, it is good to recognise what is known and what is not and be honest about this. Airway reflexes are maintained during minimal and moderate sedation but lost during anaesthesia. The point at which the reflex is lost is clear. Deep sedation is expected to require the same level of care as general anaesthesia and is not practised by dentists in the United Kingdom as it is in some other parts of the world. If starvation is required then the 2-4-6 rule is appropriate (2 h for clear fluids, 4 h for breast milk and 6 h for solids) [3, 5].

Some were concerned that monitoring recommendations had changed unnecessarily with the *Standards* publication, and in particular the requirement to measure blood pressure during the sedation. It was clear that for inhalation sedation with nitrous oxide and oxygen, clinical monitoring would be adequate. However, there was now an expectation to measure blood pressure during intravenous sedation. Previously blood pressure had been measured at the assessment visit and would have only been measured during the sedation if the patient was noted to have an elevated or particularly low blood pressure. This was based on the reasoning that midazolam does not adversely affect the cardiovascular system when a patient has normal blood pressure. It is not however unreasonable to measure blood pressure in all patients "at appropriate intervals during the procedure and post-operatively" [3,

5]. The time points will depend on the patient's risk and be determined by the sedationist's clinical judgment as described above.

7.5   Sedation Techniques

There has been a developing view that the most "straightforward" conscious sedation technique likely to be effective in enabling good quality dental care provider is usually the best first choice. Complicated techniques may be no more effective and associated with an increased risk of harm. This view was clearly articulated in the 2017 publication, *Commissioning Dental Services—Conscious Sedation in a Primary Care Setting. NHS England,* and concluded that, for new procurements, the only sedation technique that would be funded for children in England would be inhalation sedation using nitrous oxide and oxygen [7]. Such a decision is likely to have had little impact on the majority of service provision in England as more advanced techniques in children and young people have been offered by only a few providers.

The same publication also made clear that when tendering for new sedation services, it will be incumbent on the commissioners to ensure that they have appropriate clinical advice and support to advise on the clinical aspects of any bid. A commitment to clinical involvement is valued and important.

Advanced sedation techniques are defined as those for a child, young person or adult, using multiple drugs and/or anaesthetic drugs (opioid plus midazolam, ketamine, propofol, midazolam plus propofol), sevoflurane, or sevoflurane plus nitrous oxide/oxygen inhalation. When midazolam alone is used for a child then this is also described as an advanced technique [3].

7.6   Patient Pathways and Commissioning

A further recent change in the provision of conscious sedation is the development of "patient pathways". This is very much a UK innovation and has been driven by the requirement for NHS cost-effectiveness but also to develop consistent care across England with enhanced quality. The first "patient journey" was described in the *Guide for Commissioning Oral Surgery and Oral Medicine* published by NHS England in 2015. Some parts of England have moved towards incorporating electronic referral management systems to facilitate specialist referral from the general dental practitioner to dental specialist services such as oral surgery.

As this has happened some areas have also incorporated the IOSN into the referral system. This is not necessarily essential and can actually lead to a "tick-box" mentality rather than a more thoughtful use of the tool. However, it can encourage more equitable decision-making for patients and be a helpful justification for the need for conscious sedation for dental care.

Table 7.1 Minimum dataset recommended for recording the pre-sedation assessment

Scottish Dental Clinical Effectiveness Programme (SDCEP), Conscious Sedation in Dentistry—Dental Clinical Guidance Third Edition 2017

- A fully recorded medical history (including prescribed and non-prescribed drugs and any known allergies)
- ASA status
- A dental history
- A social history
- Any relevant conscious sedation and general anaesthetic history
- The dental treatment plan proposed
- Assessment of anxiety or sedation need and any tools used
- Any individual patient requirements
- Provider must not accept patients which have self-referred or who have been referred outside of the agreed local referral management processes

Referral systems can also be useful in encouraging the development of minimum datasets for information to make the best referral decisions for the patient and also to encourage dental clinicians who do not offer sedation techniques themselves to consider referral, and so not deny their patient this aspect of clinical care. A minimum dataset is likely to include some or all of the following items which are some of those recommended for recording the pre-sedation assessment by the SDCEP document as described in Table 7.1.

The document *Commissioning Dental Services: Service Standards for Conscious Sedation in a Primary Care Setting* explains that when tendering for new sedation services, it will be incumbent on the commissioners to ensure that they have appropriate clinical advice and support to advise on the clinical aspects of any bid. This advice should be from a clinical colleague who is an experienced sedationist. The document describes the minimum service specification that any new sedation provider must comply with and includes suggested patient-reported outcome measures (PROMs) and patient-reported experience measures (PREMs) as in Table 7.2. The publication like many contemporary service documents emphasises the importance of understanding the population need rather than demand and refers to the IOSN in providing evidence for this. The premise of the IOSN is that the patients' general health, behaviour and treatment complexity are taken into account alongside dental anxiety. This is the latest in a long list of conscious sedation publications and is a helpful service standard to support commissioners in the implementation and monitoring of contemporaneous conscious sedation practice in England but is likely to be looked at more widely.

It would be helpful if the use of conscious sedation was better understood but this is difficult as it is provided on a private basis as well as within NHS. There is also a current lack of consistency in the secondary care hospital system with the coding of procedures and use of conscious sedation, with different interpretations of outpatient attendance by some trusts and day-case procedures by others.

Table 7.2 Patient reported outcome measures (PROMs) and patient reported experience measures (PREMs)

Commissioning Dental Services: Service Standards for Conscious Sedation in a Primary Care Setting. NHS England. 2017
PROMs
• Was the sedation you received adequate for you to receive your dental treatment comfortably?
PREMs
• Thinking about the procedure you have had were you provided with sufficient information prior to the procedure that enabled you to understand what would happen?
• Were you and your escort provided with sufficient information to be confident in looking after you in the recovery period since your sedation?

7.7 Summary

Conscious sedation is an essential requirement for some patients to enable dental treatment to be undertaken. Selecting the appropriate patients is key to good clinical practice and dependant on clinical training and enhanced by experience. The IOSN is useful in training but also in population needs assessment to provide evidence of sedation service requirements. Clinical guidance has been recently updated with a number of publications providing detailed and helpful information on all aspects of conscious sedation practice. Clinical decision-making should be without bias and clinical practice should be evidence-based. This means that clinical judgment is required to risk assessment for individual patients to determine their best and safest care, such as the advice they are given as to whether or not they should be starved from food and fluids as part of their preoperative preparation for a sedation technique.

Paul Coulthard was Chair of the working group that published, NHS Commissioning Dental Services—Conscious Sedation in a Primary Care Setting for NHS England, and a member of the working group publishing Conscious Sedation in Dentistry—Dental Clinical Guidance, Third Edition for the Scottish Dental Clinical Effectiveness Programme (SDCEP).

References

1. Goodwin M, Pretty IA. Estimating the need for dental sedation. Paper 3. Analysis of factors contributing to non attendance for dental treatment in the general population across 12 English primary care trusts. Br Dent J. 2011;211(12):599–603.
2. Coulthard P. Oral surgery need for sedation. Editorial. Oral Surg. 2017;10(2):65–6.
3. Standards for Conscious Sedation in the Provision of Dental Care: Report of the intercollegiate Advisory Committee for Sedation in Dentistry (IACSD). 2015.
4. Coulthard P. The indicator of sedation need. SAAD Dig. 2012;28:9–12.

5. Scottish Dental Clinical Effectiveness Programme (SDCEP). Conscious sedation in dentistry - dental clinical guidance. 3rd ed. Scottish Dental Clinical Effectiveness Programme (SDCEP); 2017.
6. Coulthard P. The indicator of sedation need (IOSN). Dent Update. 2013;40(6):466–8.
7. NHS England. Commissioning dental services: service standards for conscious sedation in a primary care setting. London: NHS England; 2017.
8. Coulthard P. Issues for commissioning conscious sedation for Oral surgery. Faculty Dent J. 2013;4(2):74–9.
9. Coulthard P, Bridgman C, Gough L, Longman L, Pretty IA, Jenner T. Estimating the need for dental sedation. 1. The indicator of Sedation Need (IOSN) - a novel assessment tool. Br Dent J. 2011;211(5):E10.
10. Pretty IA, Goodwin M, Coulthard P, Bridgman C, Gough L, Sharif MO. Estimating the need for dental sedation. 2. Using IOSN as a health needs assessment tool. Br Dent J. 2011;211(5):E11.
11. Goodwin M, Coulthard P, Pretty IA, Bridgeman C, Gough L, Sharif MO. Estimating the need for dental sedation. 4. Using IOSN as a referral tool. Br Dent J. 2012;212(5):E9.

Perioperative Surgical Pain Management

8

Nadine Khawaja

Learning Objectives

- To describe the mechanisms underlying the pain experience.
- To understand the impact of perioperative pain and associated barriers.
- To discuss prescribing analgesics.
- To understand contraindication to analgesic prescribing and side effects.

Pain during and following surgery continues to be under-managed [1]. The International Association for the Study of Pain (IASP) defines post-surgical pain as a "compilation of several unpleasant sensory, emotional and mental experiences, associated with autonomic, endocrine-metabolic, physiological and behavioural responses". The continued under-management of postsurgical pain worldwide led IASP to assign 2017 as the Global Year Against Pain After Surgery [2].

8.1 Acute Pain Mechanisms

In 2011, IASP defined acute pain as "an awareness of noxious signaling from recently damaged tissue, complicated by sensitisation in the periphery and within the central nervous system". Following surgical tissue damage, multiple inflammatory mediators are released by the damaged tissue, inflammatory cells and nerves.

This "inflammatory soup" of chemical mediators (including cytokines, prostanoids (prostaglandin)), initiates the sensitisation of high-threshold nociceptors,

---

This article may contain repetition when read in conjunction with other articles in this issue as they are designed to be read independently.

N. Khawaja (✉)
Faculty of Dentistry, Oral & Craniofacial Sciences, King's College London, London, UK
e-mail: Nadine.Khawaja@Kcl.ac.uk

Table 8.1 Barriers to effective pain management

Clinician perception
- Normal result of surgery, which will resolve
- Patient's responsibility to manage
- Lack of pain protocols
- Fear of prescribing: side effects, drug interaction

Patient perception
- Normal result of surgery, which will resolve
- Stoic, not wanting to appear "fussy"/weak
- Lack of education about over-the-counter analgesics
- Fear of side effects, drug interaction, addiction
- Compliance

resulting in peripheral sensitisation [3]. This sensitisation forms an area of "primary hyperalgesia" immediately surrounding the injured area, which has a heightened response to mechanical and thermal stimuli (hyperalgesia, allodynia) [4]. There are also changes in the central processing of sensory information in the spinal cord and brain through central sensitisation and synaptic plasticity, increasing pain intensity [5]. This results in "secondary hyperalgesia" of the uninjured area of tissue that surrounds the region of primary hyperalgesia in the surgical site [3, 6].

Pain is often described as a biopsychosocial phenomenon; a multidimensional, subjective experience influenced by biological, psychological and social factors and not simply the amount of nociceptive input [7]. The emotional and cognitive components of pain are frequently as important as the afferent sensory input in determining the overall pain experience. Patients attending the dentist will experience an element of anxiety and expectation of pain, further complicating effective pain management.

There are several effective analgesics available over the counter to treat dental pain [8], however, several barriers prevent effective pain management (see Table 8.1). Changing patient and clinician attitudes to pain and analgesics through education is integral to the delivery of optimum dental care. In the primary care setting, patients may be prescribed analgesics, given analgesics (e.g. a pack of ibuprofen) or advised which analgesics to purchase.

Uncontrolled post-surgical pain causes unnecessary suffering for patients, impacting their healing, sleep, anxiety levels, stress response, attendance at work and risk of transition to chronic pain (Table 8.2) [9]. Pain and anxiety are inextricably linked. Modern-day analgesic regimens using multi-model analgesia can help reduce the negative effects of under-treated acute postsurgical pain, its sequelae and associated NHS costs [9].

8.2   Over-the-Counter Analgesics: Are They Good Enough?

The decision of which analgesics to prescribe is based on anticipated pain levels, analgesic efficacy and medical considerations (contraindications/tolerance/allergies/drug interactions), which will be discussed subsequently.

Local anaesthesia provides excellent intraoperative pain control and is discussed in another article in this issue.

Table 8.2   Sequelae of under-managed pain

Clinical perspective
- Delayed wound healing
- Increased risk of maintaining or transitioning to chronic pain
- Sustained hyperadrenergic stress response with hypertension

Patient perspective
- Suffering, loss of sleep, fear, anxiety
- Increased time off work
- Prolonged recovery of normal function and lifestyle, reducing the quality of life
- Reduced quality of life during recovery

Administrative perspective
- Increased frequency of follow-up appointments or length of stay in the hospital
- Higher complication rates and associated costs
- Increased risk of chronic pain development with consequent health care costs
- The implication that poor pain control means poor quality of surgery/care

Adapted from the 2017 IASP Global Year Against Pain After Surgery [32]

8.3   Pain Levels

Dental extractions and endodontic treatment can result in considerable postoperative pain [10]. Pain following lower third molar surgery removal has been reported to range from mild to severe [10, 11]. Post-endodontic pain has been reported to present in up to 47.3% of cases following root canal treatment (RCT) [12]. Moreover, it has been estimated that up to 10% of patients experience persistent tooth pain (over 6 months) after RCT [13, 14].

The presence/intensity of post-operative pain is dependent on several variables, including the presence and duration of pre-operative pain [12, 14–16], highlighting peripheral as well as central sensitisation during the acute pain experience. Hence, optimising analgesic interventions both before and after surgical interventions is important to reduce the risk of developing chronic pain.

Endodontic pain (irreversible pulpitis, acute apical periodontitis) has been reported to represent over 60% of all emergency dental visits [17, 18], requiring either endodontic treatment or extraction. It is suggested, therefore, that pain management for these patients is more aggressive than for patients who are booked in for elective treatment (and less likely to present with ongoing pain).

8.4   Analgesic Efficacy

Clinical pain reduction following third molar surgery has been reported to be successful if there is a relative reduction in pain >50% or absolute pain reduction of >2.5 cm on the visual analogue scale (pain intensity scale ranging from 0 = no pain to 10 = worst pain imaginable) [19].

Analgesic league tables have been used by medical and dental professionals worldwide as a guide to the relative efficacy of analgesics [20], as seen in Table 8.3. The table uses calculations of the number needed to treat (NNT) (the number of patients that need to be treated with the analgesic for one to benefit compared with

Table 8.3 Oxford league table of analgesic efficacy [20]

Analgesic and dose (mg)		
Ibuprofen + paracetamol 400+1000	▪	The number of patients who need to receive the analgesic for one to achieve at least 50% relief of pain compared with a placebo over a 6-h treatment period. The more effective the analgesic, the lower the NNT
Ibuprofen + paracetamol 200+500	▪	
Etoricoxib 120	▪	
Paracetamol + oxycodone 800/1000+10	▪	
Diclofenac potassium 100	▪	
Ketoprofen 25		
Diclofenac potassium 50	▪	
Diflunisa 1000	▪	
Ibuprofen + caffeine 200+100	▪	Single dose analgesics for moderate to severe acute pain: NNT* for at least 50% maximum pain relief over four to six hours
Ibuprofen fast acting 200	▪	
Ibuprofen fast acting 400	▪	
Ketoprofen 100	▪	
Ibuprofen + codeine 400+26/60	▪	
Paracetamol + codeine 800/1000+60	▪	
Dipyrone 500	▪	
Ibuprofen + oxycodone 400+5	▪	*NNT (number needed to treat). The number of patients needed to be treated for one to benefit compared with a control. A treatment that works for everyone, and where no patient has a response with control would have a NNT of 1. The higher the NNT, the less effective the treatment. Treatments with NNTs of 2-5 are considered effective for acute pain
Diclofenac fast acting 50	▪	
Diclofenac potassium 25	▪	
Ibuprofen + caffeine 100+100	▪	
Ketoprofen 12.5	▪	
Flurbiprofen 100	▪	
Ibuprofen acid 400	▪	
Diflunisal 500	▪	
Flurbiprofen 50	▪	
Naproxen 500/550	▪	
Paracetamol + oxycodone 600/650+10	▪	
Aspirin 1200	▪	
Ibuprofen acid 600	▪	
Naproxen 400/440	▪	
Piroxicam 20	▪	
MORPHINE 10 IM	▪	
Etodolac 400	▪	
Ibuprofen acid 200	▪	
Dexketoprofen 20/25	▪	
Flurbiprofen 25	▪	
Ketoprofen 50	▪	
Paracetamol 500	▪	
Dexketoprofen 10/12.5	▪	
Paracetamol 975/1000	▪	
Paracetamol +codeine 600/650+60	▪	
Aspirin 1000	▪	
Aspirin 600/650	▪	
Ibuprofen acid 100	▪	
Paracetamol + dextropropoxyphene 600+65	▪	
Tramadol 100	▪	
Paracetamol 600/650	▪	
Etodolac 100	▪	

NNT for at least 50% pain relief (95% CI)

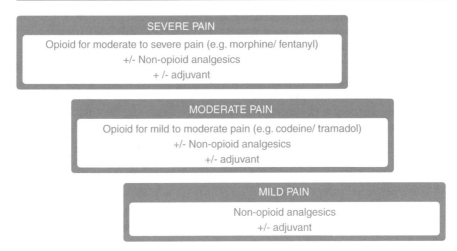

SEVERE PAIN
Opioid for moderate to severe pain (e.g. morphine/ fentanyl)
+/- Non-opioid analgesics
+ /- adjuvant

MODERATE PAIN
Opioid for mild to moderate pain (e.g. codeine/ tramadol)
+/- Non-opioid analgesics
+/- adjuvant

MILD PAIN
Non-opioid analgesics
+/- adjuvant

Fig. 8.1 World Health Organization analgesic pain ladder [22]

a control (placebo)), [21], to rank analgesics by efficacy. The surgical removal of mandibular third molars is the most common acute pain model used in trials to calculate the NNT. It may, therefore, be said that the table is particularly relevant for the management of dental pain.

The World Health Organization (WHO) analgesic ladder, for the management of differing pain severity, was introduced by the WHO in 1986 to assist analgesic prescribing for cancer patients [22] (Fig. 8.1).

Its use is still highly relevant today, being used for the management of acute and chronic pain. It makes five main recommendations:

- The combination of non-opioid analgesics (paracetamol and nonsteroidal anti-inflammatory drugs (NSAIDs)) is the backbone of pain management with the introduction of mild opioid analgesia and then stronger opioids only if the pain worsens [22]. This principle of multimodal analgesia highlights that the gold standard of pain management is by combinations of drugs, thereby maximising analgesic efficacy at lower doses and minimising side effects.
- Regular administration of analgesics (every 4–6 h) rather than "on-demand".
- Oral administration of analgesics, if possible.
- The dosage of analgesic tailored to the individual.
- Provision of detailed patient information on how to take the drug, including dosage and intervals.
- Regular reassessment of pain levels.

8.5 Non-opioid Analgesia

Paracetamol and ibuprofen are the most commonly used analgesics in acute pain management [23, 24]. Systematic reviews have demonstrated that ibuprofen (ibuprofen 400 mg NNT = 2.5) and paracetamol (paracetamol 1 g NNT = 3.8) are both effective analgesics following third molar surgery [25, 26] and post-endodontic pain [27–29]. Whilst ibuprofen has been shown to be a superior analgesic to paracetamol [30], combinations of both drugs have been shown to be more effective than either drug alone in the management of post-endodontic acute pain and following the removal of lower wisdom teeth [24, 27, 31].

NSAIDs reversibly inhibit cyclooxygenase-1 (COX-1) and cyclooxygenase-2 (COX-2) isoenzymes and, hence, prostaglandin synthesis via the arachidonic acid cascade (see Fig. 8.2) [29]. This reduction in PG, decreases inflammation, nociception and pyrexia. By decreasing inflammation, there will also be less peripheral and central sensitisation and hence, the peripheral and central nervous system will respond less to noxious stimuli.

Ibuprofen is the most commonly used NSAID in the management of inflammatory dental pain [34]. It has been shown to have a ceiling effect of 400 mg/dose, that is, doses above this are not likely to have any analgesic advantage (but may have increased anti-inflammatory effects) [35, 36]. NSAIDs are broadly classified as non-selective cyclooxygenase (COX) 1, 2 enzyme inhibitors (ibuprofen, diclofenac, aspirin) or selective COX-2 enzyme inhibitors (celecoxib, rofecoxib).

Dental pain studies have shown a strong relationship between speed of onset of pain relief and overall pain experience (maximum total pain relief) up to 6 h post-administration [37]. New fast-acting formulations of ibuprofen, using salts of ibuprofen (lysinate, arginine and sodium salts), have been introduced onto the market and show improvements in the onset of analgesia and efficacy [37]. These salts have increased water solubility and, hence, absorption of the drug. Ibuprofen salts are reported to have a Tmax (time to peak plasma concentration) before 40 min of being

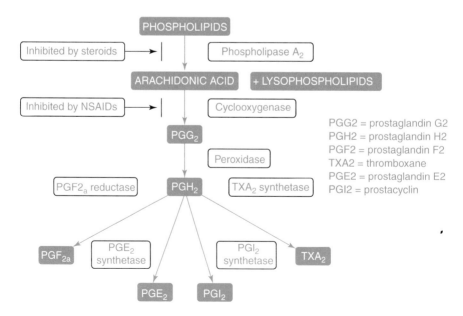

Fig. 8.2 Schematic of arachidonic acid metabolism. (Taken from Anderson [33])

administered ($p < 0.0001$) compared to standard ibuprofen formulations, which is commonly 90 min post-administration. As the level of pain intensity is proportional to the measured serum concentration of the drug [36], this faster absorption results in quicker initial pain reduction [37].

Rapid-acting analgesia has been shown to be associated with improved overall pain relief and reduced need for analgesic re-medication [37]. Importantly, the improved analgesic performance of ibuprofen salts does not also appear to produce higher rates of adverse events. In fact, dental pain studies have shown 200 mg of fast-acting ibuprofen (NNT = 2.1; 95% CI 1.9–2.4) to be as effective or better than 400 mg standard ibuprofen (NNT = 2.4; 95% CI 2.2–2.5), with a faster onset of analgesia [37]. Therefore, if lower effective doses of ibuprofen salts may be used, there is likely to be fewer adverse events. These ibuprofen salts are now commonly available over the counter and so it is suggested that they are considered as recommended dental pain relief to patients.

In the treatment of acute postoperative dental pain (uncomplicated oral surgery and endodontic procedures), ibuprofen is commonly only used for a short duration and, therefore, has reduced risks of adverse events compared to its use in the treatment of chronic inflammatory pain conditions, for example, arthritis [29]. The side effects of NSAIDs increase with a daily dose, duration of use and age (>70 years) [29]. As prostaglandins also maintain gastric protection, gastrointestinal injury is a common side effect of NSAIDs and includes gastritis, peptic ulceration, perforations and bleeding [38] (see Fig. 8.2). As a result, NSAIDs are contraindicated in patients with a history of gastrointestinal conditions including; chronic gastroesophageal reflux, peptic ulceration and gastrointestinal erosions. Moreover, reduction of thromboxane A2, through inhibition of COX-1, affects platelet aggregation and, therefore, contraindicates NSAID use in patients on anticoagulant therapy or with bleeding disorders. NSAIDs are also contraindicated in patients with renal impairment, patients at risk of arterial thrombotic event or patients with cardiac failure as renal prostaglandins and prostacyclin (needed in vasodilatation) are also synthesised by COX enzymes [38]. Recent studies have shown that the use of nonselective NSAIDs diclofenac and ibuprofen carry significant cardiovascular health risks compared with naproxen, COX-2 selective NSAIDs, paracetamol or placebo [39, 40]. Paracetamol may be used as a safe alternative in at-risk patients, as well for asthmatic patients who are sensitive to NSAIDs [41, 42].

COX-2 selective nonsteroidal anti-inflammatory drugs (NSAIDs) (coxibs) have a similar analgesic efficacy to nonselective NSAIDs, with reduced associated side effects [43]. Coxibs have been shown to have fewer gastrointestinal [44], bleeding [45] and respiratory complications [46]. Whilst concerns about cardiovascular adverse events of coxibs were identified with the use of rofecoxib (leading to its withdrawal in 2004) [47] celecoxib, which has been shown to be effective in postoperative pain following oral surgery [48, 49], has been shown to be as safe as ibuprofen or naproxen [50].

Paracetamol is a safe drug that continues to be widely used as a single agent or as part of combination drug therapy, e.g. with ibuprofen or codeine. Although the efficacy of paracetamol is well established, its mode of action is still poorly understood [33]. There is growing evidence that paracetamol has both central and peripheral mechanisms of action [51, 52].

8.6   Muiti-modal Analagesia

Paracetamol should be used in combination with NSAIDs, when possible, as they provide greater analgesia than when used alone, decreasing the effective dose and, hence, possible associated adverse effects [43]. This synergistic analgesic effect is attributed to different sites of action of the two analgesics [36]. It is suggested that adjusting the analgesic regime when the patient's pain decreases will help prevent potential side effects. For example, dose reduction of ibuprofen or taking paracetamol regularly and "topping up" with NSAIDs only when necessary.

Caffeine has also been reported to be an effective analgesic adjuvant. Ibuprofen/caffeine 400/100 mg has been shown to be superior to ibuprofen 400 mg only, for treating moderate to severe dental pain after third molar extraction [53]. An average cup of coffee contains 90 mg of caffeine.

8.7   Opioid Analgesia?

Opioid analgesics, by binding to specific opioid receptors in the central nervous system (CNS), cause reduced pain perception but also the undesirable effects of drowsiness, gastrointestinal symptoms (nausea, vomiting, constipation), respiratory depression, tolerance and addiction. On this basis, opioids should not be the first choice for the management of mild to moderate acute dental pain. They should be used only in combination with single, non-opioid analgesics (e.g. ibuprofen or paracetamol) for the management of cases of severe dental pain that are unresponsive to non-opioid multi-modal analgesia or where NSAIDs are contraindicated. In an attempt to manage the "opioid epidemic" in the United States of America, guidance to general dental practitioners has been issued, including the need to risk assess patients and identify chronic opioid users [54]. Interestingly, a recent trial demonstrated that codeine 60 mg did not improve postsurgical pain after third molar surgery, when added to ibuprofen/paracetamol 400 mg/1 g combination [55].

8.8   Preventive Analgesia

Pre-emptive/preventive analgesia presents a relatively novel approach for improving dental pain control [56]. It is defined as an anti-nociceptive treatment that is administered preoperatively, reducing the physiological consequences of induced nociceptive transmission during and after surgery. It is primarily targeted at preventing peripheral and central sensitisation, to avoid/reduce the postoperative amplification of the pain sensation, including persistent postoperative pain [57]. Local anaesthesia acts as a pre-emptive analgesic by preventing the afferent nociceptive signals and the onset of central sensitisation prior to and up to 3 h post-surgery.

Studies have shown that preoperative administration of ibuprofen can increase the success rate of inferior alveolar nerve blocks in patients with irreversible pulpitis [58, 59]. A recent study also demonstrated that preoperatively administered

Table 8.4 Adjuncts to pain management

Encourage placebo, limit nocebo
- Prescribe analgesics
- Guide expectations of analgesic efficacy
- Encourage compliance—regular dosing

Reduce anxiety and fear of the unknown
- Guide patient's expectations
- Patient contact
  - Telephone review
  - Contact details 24/7

Improve compliance and awareness
- Written post-operative patient analgesic instructions

intravenous (IV) ibuprofen reduced postoperative pain levels and rescue medication compared to preoperative IV paracetamol following lower third molar surgery [60].

8.9   Prescribing Analgesia in Practice

Table 8.4 summarises important adjunctive management of acute postoperative dental pain, which is often overlooked. Educating patients about pain control through effective communication, can improve compliance (regular analgesic administration at correct timings), guide expectations, increase the placebo and minimise the nocebo effect. Postoperative patient instruction leaflets, with information about the prescribed postoperative analgesic regime, are a useful strategy in optimising pain management in primary care.

8.10   Conclusion

Acute dental pain management is essential to the delivery of optimal dental care. A multi-modal approach, using non-opioid analgesics is the mainstay of effective acute dental pain management.

References

1. Wu CL, Raja SN. Treatment of acute postoperative pain. Lancet (London, England). 2011;377(9784):2215–25.
2. IASP. Global year against pain after surgery 2017. Available from: http://www.iasp-pain.org/GlobalYear/AfterSurgery.
3. Dawes J AD, Bennett D, Bevin S, McMahon S. Inflammatory mediators and modulators of pain. In: McMahon S, Koltzenburg M, Tracey I, Turk D, editor. Wall and Melzack's textbook of pain. Elsevier, Philadelphia, PA 2013.
4. Hudspith MJ, Sidall PJ, Munglani R. Physiology of pain. In: Hemmings HCH, Hopkins P, editors. Foundations of anesthesia: basic sciences for clinical practice. 2nd ed. London: Mosby Elsevier; 2005.

5. Vandermeulen EP, Brennan TJ. Alterations in ascending dorsal horn neurons by a surgical incision in the rat foot. Anesthesiology. 2000;93(5):1294–302; discussion 6A.

6. Juhl GI, Jensen TS, Norholt SE, Svensson P. Central sensitization phenomena after third molar surgery: a quantitative sensory testing study. Eur J Pain. 2008;12(1):116–27.

7. Gatchel RJ, Peng YB, Peters ML, Fuchs PN, Turk DC. The biopsychosocial approach to chronic pain: scientific advances and future directions. Psychol Bull. 2007;133(4): 581–624.

8. Khawaja N, Renton T. Pain Part 3: Acute orofacial pain. Dental Update. 2015;42(5):442–4, 7–50, 53–7 passim.

9. Buvanendran A-N. Fact Sheet No. 2. Pain after surgery: what health-care professionals should know. International Association for the Study of Pain (IASP); 2017.

10. Szmyd L, Shannon IL, Mohnac AM. Control of postoperative sequelae in impacted third molar surgery. J Oral Ther Pharmacol. 1965;1:491–6.

11. Howard MA, Krause K, Khawaja N, Massat N, Zelaya F, Schumann G, et al. Beyond patient reported pain: perfusion magnetic resonance imaging demonstrates reproducible cerebral representation of ongoing post-surgical pain. PLoS One. 2011;6(2):e17096.

12. Arias A, de la Macorra JC, Hidalgo JJ, Azabal M. Predictive models of pain following root canal treatment: a prospective clinical study. Int Endod J. 2013;46(8):784–93.

13. Vena DA, Collie D, Wu H, Gibbs JL, Broder HL, Curro FA, et al. Prevalence of persistent pain 3 to 5 years post primary root canal therapy and its impact on oral health-related quality of life: PEARL Network findings. J Endod. 2014;40(12):1917–21.

14. Nixdorf DR, Law AS, Lindquist K, Reams GJ, Cole E, Kanter K, et al. Frequency, impact, and predictors of persistent pain after root canal treatment: a national dental PBRN study. Pain. 2016;157(1):159–65.

15. Ince B, Ercan E, Dalli M, Dulgergil CT, Zorba YO, Colak H. Incidence of postoperative pain after single-and multi-visit endodontic treatment in teeth with vital and non-vital pulp. Eur J Dent. 2009;3(4):273–9.

16. Polycarpou N, Ng YL, Canavan D, Moles DR, Gulabivala K. Prevalence of persistent pain after endodontic treatment and factors affecting its occurrence in cases with complete radiographic healing. Int Endod J. 2005;38(3):169–78.

17. Estrela C, Guedes OA, Silva JA, Leles CR, Estrela CR, Pecora JD. Diagnostic and clinical factors associated with pulpal and periapical pain. Braz Dent J. 2011;22(4):306–11.

18. Cachovan G, Phark JH, Schon G, Pohlenz P, Platzer U. Odontogenic infections: an 8-year epidemiologic analysis in a dental emergency outpatient care unit. Acta Odontol Scand. 2013;71(3–4):518–24.

19. Martin WJ, Ashton-James CE, Skorpil NE, Heymans MW, Forouzanfar T. What constitutes a clinically important pain reduction in patients after third molar surgery? Pain Res Manag. 2013;18(6):319–22.

20. Bandolier. Bandolier Oxford league table of analgesic efficacy. 2007a.

21. Bandolier. Acute Pain. Bandolier Extra, Evidence based healthcare [Online]. 2003. Available: http://www.bandolier.org.uk/Extraforbando/APain.pdf.

22. Vargas-Schaffer G. Is the WHO analgesic ladder still valid? Twenty-four years of experience. Can Fam Physician. 2010;56(6):514–7, e202–5

23. Toms L, Derry S, Moore RA, McQua HJ. Single dose oral paracetamol (acetaminophen) with codeine for postoperative pain in adults. Cochrane Database Syst Rev. 2009;(1):Cd001547.

24. Derry S, Wiffen PJ, Moore RA. Single dose oral ibuprofen plus caffeine for acute postoperative pain in adults. Cochrane Database Syst Rev. 2015;(7):Cd011509.

25. Bandolier. Oxford League Table of Analgesia, 2007. http://www.bandolier.org.uk/booth/painpag/Acutrev/Analgesics/lftab.html.

26. Hersh EV, Levin LM, Cooper SA, Doyle G, Waksman J, Wedell D, et al. Ibuprofen liquigel for oral surgery pain. Clin Ther. 2000;22(11):1306–18.

27. Elzaki WM, Abubakr NH, Ziada HM, Ibrahim YE. Double-blind randomized placebo-controlled clinical trial of efficiency of nonsteroidal anti-inflammatory drugs in the control of post-endodontic pain. J Endod. 2016;42(6):835–42.

28. Smith EA, Marshall JG, Selph SS, Barker DR, Sedgley CM. Nonsteroidal anti-inflammatory drugs for managing postoperative endodontic pain in patients who present with preoperative pain: a systematic review and metaanalysis. J Endod. 2017;43(1):7–15.
29. Day RO, Graham GG. Nonsteroidal anti-inflammatory drugs (NSAIDs). BMJ (Clinical research ed). 2013;346:f3195.
30. Bailey E, Worthington HV, van Wijk A, Yates JM, Coulthard P, Afzal Z. Ibuprofen and/or paracetamol (acetaminophen) for pain relief after surgical removal of lower wisdom teeth. Cochrane Database Syst Rev. 2013;(12):Cd004624.
31. Moore PA, Hersh EV. Combining ibuprofen and acetaminophen for acute pain management after third-molar extractions: translating clinical research to dental practice. J Am Dental Assoc. 2013;144(8):898–908.
32. IASP. Fact Sheet No. 2. Pain after surgery: what health-care professionals should know. 2017.
33. Anderson BJ. Paracetamol (acetaminophen): mechanisms of action. Paediatr Anaesth. 2008;18(10):915–21.
34. Poveda Roda R, Bagan JV, Jimenez Soriano Y, Gallud Romero L. Use of nonsteroidal antiin-flammatory drugs in dental practice. A review. Medicina Oral, Patologia Oral y Cirugia Bucal. 2007;12(1):E10–8.
35. Seymour RA, Ward-Booth P, Kelly PJ. Evaluation of different doses of soluble ibuprofen and ibuprofen tablets in postoperative dental pain. Br J Oral Maxillofac Surg. 1996;34(1):110–4.
36. Laska EM, Sunshine A, Marrero I, Olson N, Siegel C, McCormick N. The correlation between blood levels of ibuprofen and clinical analgesic response. Clin Pharmacol Ther. 1986;40(1):1–7.
37. Moore RA, Derry S, Straube S, Ireson-Paine J, Wiffen PJ. Faster, higher, stronger? Evidence for formulation and efficacy for ibuprofen in acute pain. Pain. 2014;155(1):14–21.
38. Bhala N, Emberson J, Merhi A, Abramson S, Arber N, Baron JA, et al. Vascular and upper gastrointestinc effects of non-steroidal anti-inflammatory drugs: meta-analyses of individual participant data from randomised trials. Lancet (London, England). 2013;382(9894): 769–79.
39. Sondergaard KB, Weeke P, Wissenberg M, Schjerning Olsen AM, Fosbol EL, Lippert FK, et al. Non-steroidal anti-inflammatory drug use is associated with increased risk of out-of-hospital cardiac arrest: a nationwide case-time-control study. European heart journal Cardiovascular pharmacotherapy. 2017;3(2):100–7.
40. Schmidt M, Sorensen HT, Pedersen L. Diclofenac use and cardiovascular risks: series of nationwide cohort studies. BMJ. 2018;362:k3426.
41. Jenkins C, Costello J, Hodge L. Systematic review of prevalence of aspirin induced asthma and its implications for clinical practice. BMJ. 2004;328(7437):434.
42. Szczeklik A, Nizankowska E, Mastalerz L, Szabo Z. Analgesics and asthma. Am J Ther. 2002;9(3):233–43.
43. Moore RA, Derry S, McQuay HJ, Wiffen PJ. Single dose oral analgesics for acute postoperative pain in adults. Cochrane Database Syst Rev. 2011;(9):Cd008659.
44. Goldstein JL, Kivitz AJ, Verburg KM, Recker DP, Palmer RC, Kent JD. A comparison of the upper gastrointestinal mucosal effects of valdecoxib, naproxen and placebo in healthy elderly subjects. Aliment Pharmacol Ther. 2003;18(1):125–32.
45. Hegi TR, Bombeli T, Seifert B, Baumann PC, Haller U, Zalunardo MP, et al. Effect of rofe-coxib on platelet aggregation and blood loss in gynaecological and breast surgery compared with diclofenac. Br J Anaesth. 2004;92(4):523–31.
46. Morales DR, Lipworth BJ, Guthrie B, Jackson C, Donnan PT, Santiago VH. Safety risks for patients with aspirin-exacerbated respiratory disease after acute exposure to selective non-steroidal anti-inflammatory drugs and COX-2 inhibitors: meta-analysis of controlled clinical trials. J Allergy Clin Immunol. 2014;134(1):40–5.
47. Sun SX, Lee KY, Bertram CT, Goldstein JL. Withdrawal of COX-2 selective inhibitors rofe-coxib and valdecoxib: impact on NSAID and gastroprotective drug prescribing and utilization. Curr Med Res Opin. 2007;23(8):1859–66.

48. Aoki T, Ota Y, Mori Y, Otsuru M, Ota M, Kaneko A. Analgesic efficacy of celecoxib in patients after oral surgery: special reference to time to onset of analgesia and duration of analgesic effect. Oral Maxillofac Surg. 2016;20(3):265–71.
49. Hanzawa A, Handa T, Kohkita Y, Ichinohe T, Fukuda KI. A comparative study of oral analgesics for postoperative pain after minor oral surgery. Anesth Prog. 2018;65(1):24–9.
50. FDA FaDA, editor. Briefing Document: Joint Meeting of the Arthritis Advisory Committee and the Drug Safety and Risk Management Advisory Committee. April 24 and 25, 2018.
51. Khawaja N. Cerebral blood flow imaging of acute post-operative pain and analgesic response following third molar surgery. London: King's College London; 2016.
52. Pickering G, Kastler A, Macian N, Pereira B, Valabregue R, Lehericy S, et al. The brain signature of paracetamol in healthy volunteers: a double-blind randomized trial. Drug Des Dev Ther. 2015;9:3853–62.
53. Weiser T, Richter E, Hegewisch A, Muse DD, Lange R. Efficacy and safety of a fixed-dose combination of ibuprofen and caffeine in the management of moderate to severe dental pain after third molar extraction. Eur J Pain. 2018;22(1):28–38.
54. Nack B, Haas SE, Portnof J. Opioid use disorder in dental patients: the latest on how to identify, treat, refer and apply laws and regulations in your practice. Anesth Prog. 2017;64(3):178–87.
55. Best AD, De Silva RK, Thomson WM, Tong DC, Cameron CM, De Silva HL. Efficacy of codeine 5 when added to paracetamol (acetaminophen) and ibuprofen for relief of postoperative pain after surgical removal of impacted third molars: a double-blinded randomized control trial. J Oral Maxillofac Surg. 2017;75(10):2063–9.
56. Penprase B, Brunetto E, Dahmani E, Forthoffer JJ, Kapoor S. The efficacy of preemptive analgesia 5 for postoperative pain control: a systematic review of the literature. AORN J. 2015;101(1):94–105.e8.
57. Dahl JB, Kehlet H. Preventive analgesia. Curr Opin Anaesthesiol. 2011;24(3):331–8.
58. Bidar M, Mortazavi S, Forghani M, Akhlaghi S. Comparison of Effect of Oral Premedication with Ibuprofen or Dexamethasone on Anesthetic Efficacy of Inferior Alveolar Nerve Block in Patients with Irreversible Pulpitis: A Prospective, Randomized, Controlled, Double-blind Study. The Bulletin of Tokyo Dental College. 2017;58(4):231–6.
59. Nagendrababu V, Pulikkotil SJ, Veettil SK, Teerawattanapong N, Setzer FC. Effect of Nonsteroidal Anti-inflammatory Drug as an Oral Premedication on the Anesthetic Success of Inferior Alveolar Nerve Block in Treatment of Irreversible Pulpitis: A Systematic Review with Meta-analysis and Trial Sequential Analysis. J Endod. 2018;44(6):914–22.e2.
60. Viswanath A, Oreadi D, Finkelman M, Klein G, Papageorge M. Does pre-emptive administration of intravenous ibuprofen (caldolor) or intravenous acetaminophen (ofirmev) reduce postoperative pain and subsequent narcotic consumption after third molar surgery? J Oral Maxillofac Surg. 2019;77(2):262–70.
61. Weil K, Hooper L, Afzal Z, Esposito M, Worthington HV, van Wijk AJ, et al. Paracetamol for pain relief after surgical removal of lower wisdom teeth. Cochrane Database Syst Rev. 2007;(3):Cd004487.

Optimal Local Anaesthesia for Dentistry

9

Tara Renton

Learning Objectives

- To challenge the assumption that inferior dental blocks are the "go-to" local anaesthesia (LA) procedure for mandibular dentistry.
- To challenge current LA practice.
- To understand the importance of novel La agents and techniques to optimise pain management during surgery whilst minimising risks of complications.

9.1 What Is the Role of Local Anaesthesia in Managing Analgesia for Dental Patients?

Your patients want two main outcomes when they come to visit your practice: pain-free injections and painless procedures [1]. However, needles and tablets are small part of the holistic pain management in your dental patients [2]. The definition of pain is that it is "an unpleasant sensory and emotional experience associated with actual or potential tissue damage, or described in terms of such damage" [3]. The brain overlays the pain sensation on the part of your body that's getting hurt to protect it from harm. There are four types of pain [4]: two healthy and two pathological. Healthy protective pain includes firstly; nociceptive pain, which is the conversion of tissue injury and release of algogenic factors (intracellular cellular components

The original version of the chapter has been revised. Spelling errors in Table 9.7 were corrected. A correction to this chapter can be found at https://doi.org/10.1007/978-3-030-86634-1_13

This article may contain repetition when read in conjunction with other articles in this issue as they are designed to be read independently.

T. Renton (✉)
Faculty of Dentistry, Oral & Craniofacial Sciences, King's College London, London, UK
e-mail: Tara.renton@kcl.ac.uk

© The Author(s), under exclusive license to Springer Nature   101
Switzerland AG 2022, corrected publication 2023
T. Renton (ed.), *Optimal Pain Management for the Dental Team*, BDJ Clinician's
Guides, https://doi.org/10.1007/978-3-030-86634-1_9

released due to cell damage) acting as "foreign bodies" exciting pain receptors on nociceptive nerve fibres (C, A delta and A beta fibres), causing transduction from chemical inflammation into an action potential and transmission the progression of an action potential advancing up to the tertiary order neurones to the somatosensory cortex; once reached the "ouch" is acknowledged resulting in the reflex withdrawal of the digit from danger. Inflammatory pain follows nociceptive pain if tissue damage occurs promoting tissue healing. This process should usually resolve in days or weeks depending on the degrees of damage and persistent of infection.

Local anaesthesia blocks nociceptive pain very successfully, but, due to pain's multiple components, increasing evidence supports that educating patients in expected pain levels, being caring, empathetic, providing appropriate anxiolysis, distraction and on occasions providing this alone, is not enough to manage perioperative pain. Some patients may be stoic types, able to cope with the anticipated and actual surgical discomfort, whereas others may be more susceptible to lack of coping and catastrophising, needing a lot more attention. Holistic patient management is all important in pain management, including alternative techniques i.e. hypnosis and acupuncture.

The patients' expectations are paramount and we know that all patients expect pain when visiting their dentist [5]. It is important to point out to your patient that you are not a magician but a surgeon and it is impossible to do complex surgery on patients without causing some minor discomfort intraoperatively and occasionally moderate pain postoperatively. Perioperative dental pain is not managed well in dentistry and is the most common adverse event reported by dentists [6, 7] and by patients [8]. Sixty percent of a representative sample of the general population aged 15 years or older have reported pain at least once during a dental visit [9, 10].

Local anaesthetic injection plus analgesic tablets are not enough. Local anaesthesia is only a small part of operative pain management [2]. Pain and its management are complex, as the individual's pain experience is unique and based upon their gender, beliefs, religion, ethnicity, prior pain experience, psychological factors, nocebo and placebo effects, etc. [5] there are many psychological factors driving the response to acute pain related to surgery and in relation to the development of chronic postsurgical pain.

The key aspects for operative pain management include:

- Patient factors, including:
  - Managing the patients' expectations and anxiety. Education about pre and postoperative events with clear and frank two-stage consent allowing the patient some control of their treatment decisions.
  - Appropriate anxiolysis (assessment and management) will elevate pain thresholds and improve pain management.
- Medical aspects, including:
  - Optimal local anaesthetic practise.
  - Appropriately prescribed analgesics.
- Surgical factors: Good surgical practice minimises pain for the patient, including minimal access technique.
- Post-op advice with accessibility for the patient contacting the practice and/or surgeon with clear postoperative advice on mouth care maintenance and analgesics use.

9.2 How Do We Minimise Systemic Complications of Dental Local Anaesthesia?

Over one billion dental local anaesthetic injections are given annually worldwide (communication Malamed S FDI lecture 2017). The reported adverse reaction rate is 1:1,000,000 and the mortality (death) rate from dental local anaesthetic injections has been stated at 0.000002%. Allergies are very rare and can often be psychosomatic [11].

The definition of the term "adverse reaction" covers noxious and unintended effects resulting not only from the authorised use of a medicinal product at normal doses but also from medication errors and uses outside the terms of the marketing authorisation, including the misuse and abuse of the medicinal product. The range of pharmaceuticals used in dental practice is relatively small, consisting primarily of sedatives, local anaesthetics, analgesics and antibiotics. Adverse drug reactions are categorised as type A or type B.

- **Type A**: Reactions are more common and are generally attributable to known pharmacological or toxic effects of the drug.
- **Type B**: idiosyncratic, unpredictable, acute/sub-acute, not related to the known mechanism.

The most common adverse reactions to LA include:

- **Vasovagal** attack or faint. Nearly all patient-related collapses during dental LA are faints allergies. A study carried out at Dundee Dental School showed that of 27 cases of "local anaesthetic allergies", only one was caused by the anaesthetic injection (and this was a sulphite allergy, not a drug allergy) [12]. This can be overcome by good chairside manner and observation of the patient. If a prolonged procedure is anticipated the patient should have eaten prior to the procedure or be provided with a glucose drink. Any patient who is anxious must be provided with suitable anxiolysis.
- **Allergy** to local anaesthetic agents. This is very rare and usually related to adjunctive agents including a bung (latex) [13], the preservative (sodium metabisulphites), antiseptic, vasoconstrictor or, very rarely, the local anaesthetic agent. Most LA agents are now latex-free. Esters are highly allergenic and there are no documented allergy to amides. The patient is more likely to be allergic to bisulphate preservatives (needed for vasoconstricture). The least allergenic LAs are mepivacaine or plain prilocaine. Allergy is not dose-dependent, unlike toxicity [14]. The signs of allergy include breathlessness, disorientation and distress, urticaria hypotension and collapse. Immediate action is required including: call for help, 1:1000 units' epinephrine IM and provision of oxygen.
- Adverse effects usually caused by high-plasma concentration of LA drug resulting from:
  - Inadvertent intravascular injection related to block injections.
  - Excessive dose or rate of injection.

Table 9.1 Adverse effects

Adverse effects are usually caused by high plasma concentration of either local anaesthesia (LA) drug or adjunctive content resulting from
• Delayed absorption of LA
• Reduction of the systemic plasma levels of the LA
• Prolongation of the duration of action of the LA
• Reinforcement of the intensity of the LA's effects—not dependent on the concentration
• Reduction of local blood perfusion

Table 9.2 Maximum doses of local anaesthetic agents

Drug	Max dose (mg/kg)	1/10th cartridge (mg)
2% lidocaine	4.4	3.6–4.4
2% mepivacaine	4.4	4.0
3% mepivacaine	4.4	6.0
3% prilocaine	6.0	6.6
4% prilocaine	6.0	8.0
4% articaine	7.0	6.8–8.0

  – Medically compromised patients.
• Delayed drug clearance.
• Drug interactions (Table 9.1).

Adverse events happen in relation to the concentration and dose of LA. Intravascular injections are more likely to occur with block than with intraosseous and periodontal injections. Minimising risk of overdose includes avoiding:

• All four-quadrant treatments (staged treatment for elderly patients).
• Plain La (no vasoconstrictor).
• Full cartridge injections (should commonwealth move to 1.7 mL cartridges?)
• Exceeding maximum recommended dose (see Table 9.2).

Young and elderly patients must be suitably assessed for their weight. A child of 5 years weighs 18–20 kg; therefore, the maximum dose is 88 mg (2 × 2.2 mL lidocaine cartridges). Due to their size, children are at high risk of toxicity. Goodson and Moore have documented catastrophic consequences of this drug interaction in paediatric patients receiving procedural sedation, along with excessive dosages of local anesthetics [15].

Medical issues: (see Table 9.3) any health aspects that include metabolising or excreting. The main medical risks are:

• Patients with cardiovascular diseases
• Patients with endocrine diseases
• Patients with CNs disorders
• Patients with lung diseases

Table 9.3 Lidocaine toxicity

At serum levels patients may complain of

- 1–5 µg/mL
  - Tinnitus
  - Lightheadedness
  - Circumoral numbness
  - Diplopia
  - Metallic taste
  - May complain of nausea and/or vomiting, or they may become more talkative
- 5–8 µg/mL
  - Nystagmus, slurred speech, localized muscle twitching or fine tremors may be noticed. Patients also have been noted to have hallucinations at these levels
- 8–12 µg/mL
  - Focal seizure activity occurs; this can progress to generalised tonic–clonic seizures. Respiratory depression occurs at extremely high blood levels (20–25 µg/mL) and can progress to coma

Aspiration during dental La is a legal requirement in the United Kingdom. Avoiding intravascular La is possible by avoiding injection intra-vascularly by using aspiration and avoiding intraosseous injections and being aware of the increased vascularity of inflamed tissue whilst always observing clinical reactions by:

- Talking to the patient during the injection and monitor their ECG/blood pressure to realise early symptoms of central nervous and cardiovascular toxicity if they are at risk.
- Stopping the injection immediately when early symptoms are realised.
- Considering the time course for the development of toxic signs (5–10 min).
- Avoiding long-acting and potent substances (bupivacaine is the most neuro-toxic agent).

A recent survey of 2731 patients undergoing LA for dental treatment reported that 45.6% pts had medical risk factors (mostly cardiovascular). The overall LA complication rate was 4.5% complications (5.7% in risk pts) non-risk patients 3.5% which were most commonly dizziness, tachycardia, agitation, bronchospasm. Severe complications including seizures, bronchospasm occurred rarely (0.07%). Overall there were fewer complications with articaine 4% i:100 K epinephrine compared with articaine 4% i:200 K epinephrine [16].

Articaine is less toxic than lidocaine at the same concentration as it has a high binding plasma rate reducing crossing the placenta or blood–brain barrier. Metabolism of articaine occurs in tissue and plasma (rather than in the liver for lidocaine or bupivacaine) and lidocaine is only 50% degraded after 1.5–3 h–much slower than articaine, of which 50% is eliminated after 20 min.

All suspected adverse events to local anaesthesia should be reported. This can be done online via the MHRA Yellow Card website (at www.mhra.gov.uk/yellowcard) or by calling the National Yellow Card Information service on 0808 100 3352 (10 a.m. to 2 p.m. Monday–Friday). In addition, dental practices should sign up to receive MHRA alerts. Subscribe at www.gov.uk/drug-device-alerts/email-signup.

9.3   What Are the Medical Modifiers for Dental LA?

There are very few absolute medical contraindications to local anaesthetic and these are listed in Table 9.4. There are some relative but not absolute contraindications for adrenaline use including:

- Hypertension, angina pectoris, heart failure
- Diabetes mellitus
- Bronchial asthma
- Regularly taken medication (TCAs, MAO inhibitors, beta-blockers)
- Pregnancy
- Narrow-angle glaucoma

However, prudent avoidance of blocks, or aspirating when using blocks and slow injection, low dosage, staged treatments allows the use of adrenaline in patients with these conditions. Use of low dose adrenaline LA agents can be used in these cases (see Table 9.5) [16]:

- Specific systemic complications have been reported with dental local anaesthetics including Methaemoglobinemia: benzocaine should no longer be used. Prilocaine should not be used in children younger than 6 months, in pregnant women, or in patients taking other oxidising drugs. The dose should be limited to 2.5 mg/kg. At low levels (1–3%), methaemoglobinemia can be asymptomatic, but higher levels (10–40%) may be accompanied by any of the following complaints: cyanosis, breathlessness, tachycardia, fatigue and weakness [17].
- Drug interactions:
  - Lidocaine can interact with CNS depressants and with H2 blockers (PPIs).

Table 9.4 Absolute medical contraindications for LA

Include: Pheochromocytoma	Adrenaline producing tumour of the adrenal gland
Hyperthyroidism	Elevated levels of thyroxine which lead to sensitisation of adrenaline receptors
Tachycardic arrhythmias	Unstable ventricular fibrillation
Sulphite allergy	Anaphylactic reaction

Table 9.5 Low dose adrenaline LA agents can be used in these cases ideally using infiltration rather than Block, intra-osseous or intraligamental techniques

Articaine 4% with adrenaline 1:400,000	12.5 mL
Articaine 4% with adrenaline 1:200,000	8 mL
Articaine 4% with adrenaline 1:100,000	4 mL
Articaine 4% without adrenaline	7 mL
Mepivacaine 3% without adrenaline	10 mL
Mepivacaine 2% without adrenaline	15 mL

- Epinephrine:
  Propranolol is the only nonselective beta-blocker reported to have the potential to cause severe hypertension and reflex bradycardia in the presence of epinephrine.
  A significant risk does not appear to be associated with the use of epinephrine and cardioselective beta-blockers.

Many complications or adverse events arise during dental local anaesthetics due to the patient being overly anxious or not well informed. Thus, your LA technique must address several aspects including:

- Recheck medical history at every visit:
  - Patient's recent prescription chart (<2 weeks).
  - Patient's blood pressure.
  - Care with small patients:
    Children.
    Elderly (sarcopenia—the loss of muscle mass—reduces body mass significantly after 60 years).
- Good preoperative assessment of medical history and anxiety levels.
- Reassurance/warnings (avoid showing the patient the syringe).
- Give your patient a feeling of control.
- Distraction.
- Topical LA.
- Place fingertip near the region where you are about to inject.
- Warm LA cartridges.
- Slow injections are less painful and more effective [11].

A key factor in patient satisfaction is a sense that the caregiver is doing their best and is genuinely concerned that therapy is adequate [18].

9.4   How Do We Minimise Regional Complications of LA?

9.4.1   Avoiding Failed LA

There are many myths regarding failed LA in dentistry [19]. Local anaesthesia failure is often assumed to be the fault of the clinician due to the general overestimation of the effectivity of block anaesthesia providing pulpal anaesthesia in the mandible. The onset of lip numbness occurs usually within 5–9 min of injection and pulpal anaesthesia follows (15–16 min) [20–22]. Slow onset of pulpal anesthesia (after 15 min) occurs approximately 19–27% of the time in mandibular teeth and approximately 8% of patients have onset after 30 min [23]. Lip numbness does not guarantee pulpal anaesthesia and failure to achieve lip numbness occurs about 5% of the time with experienced clinicians [24–26].

Inferior dental blocks are remarkably inefficient at providing pulpal anaesthesia for dental procedures [22, 23, 27]. Malamed stated the rate of inadequate anaesthesia ranged from 31% to 81%. When expressed as success rates, this indicates a range of 19–69%. These numbers are so wide-ranging as to make the selection of a standard for the rate of success for IANB seemingly impossible [11].

There are many myths regarding failed LA in dentistry:

- Inferior dental blocks are remarkably inefficient at providing pulpal anaesthesia for dental procedures particularly in mandibular premolars, canines and incisors [11].
- Numbness (anaesthesia or "lip sign") of the patient's lip does not indicate pulpal anaesthesia.
- The optimal pulpal anaesthesia rates occur 12–15 min after an inferior dental block (IDB). (Are we waiting long enough)?
- Articaine 4% IDBs are no more efficient than lidocaine 2% IDBs and have the additional potential risk of increased nerve injury rates.
- Accuracy of injecting near the inferior alveolar nerve does not improve analgesia (therefore we should not be aiming to "stab" the nerve) [28, 29].
- Speed of IDB injection: a slow inferior alveolar nerve block injection (60 s) results in a higher success rate of pulpal anaesthesia and less pain than a rapid injection (15 s) [30].
- Pathological (infection) [31, 32]: pulpitis is a challenging clinical problem, and can only be overcome by increasing the dose of anaesthetic in the area, with increased accuracy of the placement of the anaesthetic solution [33].
- Choice of technique, insufficient dose, poor technique, damaged LA due to poor storage [34].
- Giving another inferior alveolar nerve block does not help the patient if they feel pain during operative procedures. The second injection does not provide additional anaesthesia—the first injection is just "catching up" [23].
  - Increasing the volume to two cartridges of lidocaine or increasing the epinephrine concentration from 1:100,000 to 1:50,000 will not provide better pulpal anesthesia [35, 36].
  - Using higher concentration agents for block injections is not evidenced to improve efficacy [26, 37, 38]. Specifically articaine compared with lidocaine IDBs has no or limited additional efficacy [39, 40].
  - Computed techniques do not ad advantage for IDB efficacy [41].
  - There is no evidence to support using direct or indirect Halstead IDB technique or the improved efficacy of using Gow-Gates of Akinosi techniques.

9.5   How Do We Manage Failed IDB?

- There is increasing evidence that additional injections (buccal infiltration, intraseptal, intraligamental, intraosseous) can enhance and even replace IDBs. Supplemental injections can improve mandibular pupal anaesthesia [32].

- Recent studies report that giving a buccal infiltration of a cartridge of 4% articaine with 1:100,000 epinephrine after an inferior alveolar nerve block significantly increased success (88%) when compared to a lidocaine formulation (71% success) [42, 43]. In a study of 182 patients, 122 achieved successful pulpal anaesthesia within 10 min after initial IANB injection and only 82 experienced pain-free treatment. Additional Articaine buccal infiltration (ABI) and intraosseous (IO) allowed more successful (pain-free) treatment [44].
- The addition of intraligamental injections may assist in extractions [45, 46]. However, intraligamental injections are unlikely to be as effective at IDB alone for other dental procedures.
- The addition of the intraosseous injection after an inferior alveolar nerve block, in the first molar, will provide a quick onset and a high incidence of pulpal anaesthesia (approximately 90%) for 60 min. Clinically, the supplemental intraosseous injection works very well but systemic cardiac effects are related to the "intravenous" nature of this injection [47, 48].
- Prescribing preoperative ibuprofen prior to dental treatment for pulpitic molar teeth is likely to significantly increase the effectiveness of the IDB local anaesthesia [49].

The main issues appear to be the overestimation of the efficacy of IDBs in general, impatience and lack of awareness that one must wait over 15 min for maximum efficacy of a lidocaine block, in addition to the lack of use of alternative techniques that provide improved pulpal anaesthetic rates for anterior teeth.

9.6   How Do We Minimise Regional Complications of LA?

Most of these complications can be avoided by careful technique and avoidance of intravascular injections but even when clinicians use the utmost care, by aspirating before the injection and noting anatomical landmarks, intra-arterial injections can occur during inferior alveolar nerve blocks [52]. Fortunately, permanent damage to nerves, facial and oral tissues and eyes is rare.

Possible regional complications related to IDBs include:

- Facial palsy is likely due to poor IDB technique with too deep or superior injection through the coronoid process into the sheaths of the parotid gland through which the facial nerve travels [53].
- Tissue trauma-haematoma trismus. In patients who have coagulopathies or platelet malfunction avoidance of block, injections are advisable but occasionally unavoidable.
- Fracture of the needle is more likely to occur with 30 gauge needles, using needles too short leaving no additional space between the hub and tissues and pre-bending of the needle prior to injection [54, 55].
- Ophthalmic complications [56].

Table 9.6 Risk factors for nerve injury related to dental local anaesthesia [31, 50, 51]

Block anaesthesia	59
Lingual nerve > IAN	60
Blind block injections	61–63
There is criticism of teaching the use of blind injections in dentistry	
• Technique or anatomy?	No evidence that direct Halstead causes more lingual nerve injuries than indirect technique
Concentration of LA agent	59, 60, 64–71
Speed of injection	
Multiple injections	59
Severe pain on injection	60% more likely to experience persistent neuropathy [50]
LA agent toxicity	Increasing toxicity at same concentration
	Bupivicaine > Mepivacaine > Prilocaine > Lidocaine > Articaine
• Type of vasoconstrictor?	No evidence
• Sedated GA	No evidence
• Lack LA aspiration	No evidence

- Nerve injury related to IDB injections may cause permanent neuropathy in lingual and inferior alveolar nerves often associated with combined numbness, paraesthesia and neuropathic pain. Though LA-related permanent nerve injury is rare, once the injury occurs approximately 75% may resolve but the remaining 25% is untreatable. Most patients with trigeminal nerve injuries experience chronic pain in their lip, teeth and gums or tongue and gums, depending on which nerve is damaged. This is a lifelong burden that these patients find difficult to accommodate, especially when they were never warned about the possible risk. The risk of nerve injury can be mitigated by altering the block technique or by avoiding block anaesthesia altogether. The risk factors for nerve injury related to dental anaesthesia are listed in Table 9.6.

The incidence of persistent neuropathy related to dental IDBs is rare, estimated to be between one in 14,000 temporary and one in 52,000 permanent (25% permanent), 59 1:26,762 and 1:160,571 [57], one in 27,415 cases [58], one in 785,000 injections, to one in 13,800.970 [59]. The majority of nerve injuries are painful in patients seeking care, consistent with other surgical sensory neuropathies leading to a condition known as chronic postsurgical pain. Unfortunately for these patients, the unforeseen complication of routine dental care leads to life-changing orofacial pain with subsequent significant functional and psychological sequelae.

Management: there is no evidence-based treatment for these nerve injuries—we have to sit and wait whilst caring for the patient. If pain is caused during an IDB, arrange to contact the patient the next day to exclude persistent neuropathy (pain, numbness and or altered sensation), reassure them that 75% recover, medical intervention including non-steroidal anti-inflammatory drugs (NSAIDs), vitamin B and steroids as used for spinal iatrogenic nerve injuries may be effective in reducing neural inflammation and irritation—but there is no evidence to support this, aside from patients being reassured that their clinician is trying to help them.

Should patients be warned of possible rare nerve injuries related to dental LA? Based upon the Montgomery ruling, clinicians must now ensure that patients are aware of any "material risks" involved in a proposed treatment, and of reasonable alternatives, following the judgment in the case *Montgomery v Lanarkshire Health Board*. This is a marked change to the previous "Bolam test", which asks whether a doctor's conduct would be supported by a responsible body of medical opinion.

This test will no longer apply to the issue of consent, although it will continue to be used more widely in cases involving other alleged acts of negligence. Thus, one has to question when would a permanent burning tongue or elicited neuralgic pain of the face be caused whenever eating, kissing, speaking or out in the cold, is not material to a patient? Suggested routine consent was suggested in the United States in 1939 [60]. In Germany there is already a legal precedent to warn all patients undergoing dental LA of possible nerve injury, and any patient undergoing spinal or epidural injections in the United Kingdom must warn patients of possible permanent motor or sensory nerve injuries in one in 57,000 [61].

Thus, prevention of LA nerve injuries is paramount and most effectively achieved by avoiding block anaesthesia. Dentistry is the only healthcare profession taught to aim for nerves blindly during block injections. There is increasing pressure to use ultrasound neural location to minimise systemic toxicity and nerve injuries as practiced in regional block anaesthesia elsewhere in the body. Other strategies would include avoiding risk factors (Table 9.6 [47–75]) but mainly avoid block anaesthesia and using infiltration techniques instead.

9.7   What Is Wrong with Our Current Practice and How Can We Do Better?

Proposed tailored smart LA practice:

- Technique
- Agent
- Volume

The limitations of IDB in providing swift mandibular pulpal anaesthesia are recognised and recent evidence supports the use of infiltration mandibular dentistry. Interestingly, for decades dentists have routinely undertaken maxillary dentistry with infiltrations, accepting that nerves within bone are accessible to submucosal local anaesthetic techniques. With respect to maxillary infiltration anaesthesia,

Table 9.7 Volume recommendation for maxillary local anaesthesia in dentistry

Technique	Volume (mL)
Supraperiosteal (infiltration)	0.6
Posterior superior alveolar (PSA)	0.9–1.8
Middle superior alveolar (MSA)	0.9–1.2
Anterior superior alveolar (ASA)	0.9–1.2
Anterior middle superior alveolar (AMSA)	1.4–1.8
Palatal approach-anterior superior alveolar (P-ASA)	1.4–1.8
Greater (anterior) palatine	0.45–0.6
Nasopalatine	0.45 (max)
Palatal infiltration	0.2–0.3
Maxillary (V2) nerve block	1.8

Taken from Malamed SF Techniques of maxillary anaesthesia in *Handbook of local anaesthesia* Malamed SF 6th edition Mosby Elsevier 2013, St Louis page 223 [78]

some studies have found 4% articaine to be more effective than 2% lidocaine for lateral incisors but not molars [58], while others reported no clinical superiority for this injection [72, 73]. A recent randomised controlled trial found a statistically significant difference supporting the use of 4% articaine in place of 2% lidocaine for buccal infiltration in patients experiencing irreversible pulpitis in maxillary posterior teeth [74].

As mentioned previously, nerve blocks are related to nerve injury and there are vno indications to use palatal, incisal or infraorbital nerve blocks for dentistry except in very rare exceptions; for example, spreading infection from canines or premolar use of block anaesthesia will prevent the need for general anaesthetic drainage and extractions. Several studies report the lack of indications for palatal block injections [51, 75]. There is increasing evidence that additional injections (buccal infiltration, intraseptal, intraligamental, intraosseous) can enhance and even replace IDBS [31, 34, 44, 74]. Lidocaine infiltration is likely as effective as articaine for maxillary dentistry [76]. A recent systematic review highlighted that there is no benefit in using articaine infiltration for maxillary dentistry but articaine is 3.6 more times effective than lidocaine for mandibular infiltration dentistry [77] (Table 9.7).

9.8 Can Articaine 4% Infiltration Replace Lidocaine 2% IANBs for Routine Dentistry?

Undoubtedly, using infiltration and not IDBs improves patient comfort as patients will undoubtedly prefer having full lingual sensation and shorter duration LA anaesthesia after dental treatment [31]. Not only are buccal infiltration techniques proving as or more effective than IDBs but intraligamental injections can also be used effectively for exodontia as intraligamental injections are effectively intravascular with more likely systemic effects but in addition, there is reported higher post restorative pain levels [79, 80] (Table 9.8).

Table 9.8 Volume recommendation for mandibular local anaesthesia in dentistry

Technique	Volume (mL)
Inferior alveolar (IANB)	1.5
Buccal	0.3
Gow-gates (kind of IANB)	1.8
Vazirani-Akinosi (kind of IANB)	1.5–1.8
Mental	0.6
Incisive	0.6–0.9

Taken from Malamed SF Techniques of maxillary anaesthesia in *Handbook of local anaesthesia* Malamed SF 6th edition Mosby Elsevier 2013, St Louis Page 223 [78]

9.9 IANBs Are Unnecessary to Treat the Following

- Pulpitis mandibular molars in adults [81, 82].
- Exodontia in adults and children [45, 83].
- Implant surgery: 88,120 patients requiring the placement of a single implant in order to replace a missing first mandibular were randomly allocated to two groups comparing crestal with infiltration. No nerve damage occurred using either anaesthesia type, therefore the choice of type of anaesthesia is a subjective clinical decision. However, it may be preferable to use a low dose (0.9 mL) of subperiosteal anaesthesia, since it is unnecessary to deliver 7.2 mL of articaine to anaesthetise a single mandibular molar implant site [84].
- Restorative mandibular care in kids [85]: however, a recent study of 57 paediatric patients undergoing restorative mandibular treatment reported a higher success and less painful treatment with IANB. There was no statistically significant difference in local analgesia success between articaine and lignocaine when delivered via buccal infiltration [86].

9.10 The Benefit of Computerised Systems for Infiltration Techniques

There is limited evidence to support that computerised infiltration systems are more effective but those regularly using these systems empirically report better patient acceptance and comfort during injections [87].

9.11 What Is the Best Agent?

Articaine (4-methyl-3-[2-(propylamino)-propionamido]-2-thiophene-carboxylic acid, methyl ester hydrochloride) is a unique amide LA in that it contains thiophene, instead of a benzene ring. The thiophene ring allows greater lipid solubility and potency as a greater portion of an administered dose can enter neurons. It is the only amide anaesthetic containing an ester group, allowing hydrolysation in unspecific blood esterases. About 90% of articaine metabolises quickly via hydrolysis in the blood into its inactive metabolite articaine acid, which is excreted by the kidney in the form of articaine acid glucuronide. Its metabolism is age-dependent, where clearance and volume of distribution decrease with increasing age. The elimination serum half-life of articaine is 20 min and of articaine acid, it is 64 min [88, 89]. Articaine at three different comparative lidocaine concentrations prove more effective in providing mandibular pulpal anaesthesia [90, 91]; however, articaine is 3.6 times more effective for mandibular infiltration dentistry [77] and a recent study demonstrated that 2% articaine is as effective as 4% articaine using IDB for mandibular dental extraction in adults [92, 93]. In summary, more research is needed before recommending replacing 4% with 2% articaine for all dental procedures.

The concentration of epinephrine may be reduced from one in 100 to one in 200 and equally effective for third molar extraction 100 and epinephrine concentration of one in 400 may only be required for paediatric extractions using 4% articaine [94].

So is the future agent for dental anaesthesia 2% articaine with 1:200 K–400 K epinephrine for all LA techniques and dental procedures in adults? Could we use epinephrine-free LA for paedodontic dentistry? Further research is needed.

9.12   What LA Volumes Should We Be Using?

The most common LA cartridge volume used worldwide is 1.8 mL [95]. Dentists in France and Japan use only 1 mL cartridges and the Commonwealth 2.2 mL cartridges. Dictation of LA volume to achieve effective pain control depends on the diameter of nerve and accuracy of the technique.

Infiltration techniques require significantly less LA volume compared with block techniques (0.6–9 mL), Gow-Gates only block anaesthesia technique where full cartridge 1.8–2.2 mL is recommended and infraorbital LA block requires 1.8–2.2 mL [11].

Thus the continued use of 2.2 mL cartridges should be questioned and changed to 1.8 mL cartridges, which would improve patient safety and likely impact minimally on repeated injections,

The future interest is the possibility of the development of newer improved agents (sensory blocking agents only) and devices and techniques for achieving profound sensory anesthesia. A nasal spray (http://clinicaltrials.gov/ct2/show/NCT01302483) has been shown to anesthetise maxillary anterior six teeth is set to be tested in an FDA phase 3 trial, which will assess the spray's effectiveness compared to the current "gold standard" treatment—painful anesthesia injections.

Buffering of acidic local anaesthetics to more neutral physiological pH allows for speedier LA onset and is already in use in the United States. A recent development is a syringe micro vibrator (SMV) [96], a new device being introduced in dentistry to alleviate pain and anxiety of intraoral injections.

9.13 Conclusion

Substantive evidence supports a transition from block anaesthesia to infiltration dentistry for most dental care [97–99]. A radical change in practice is required with regard to so many aspects of patient safety based upon current evidence, whilst acknowledging further research would be ideal. With the current research legislation, undertaking simple efficacy studies of existing commonly used LA agents is prohibitively expensive and unlikely to be funded by pharmaceutical companies, limiting the provision of future robust supportive research. Infiltration LA for implantology is a good example where common sense and application of optimal technique has occurred without a robust evidence base providing safer more effective patient care.

- A tailored approach to dental local anaesthesia should be recommended to prevent the continued unnecessary use of IDBs when infiltration anaesthesia is likely more effective for most dental procedures. Tailored LA is dictated by the site and procedure. See Fig. 9.1 summarising the optimal anaesthetic techniques.
- The lack of safety giving blind block injections with likely systemic and local complications (especially nerve injury) may be considered "indefensible".
- IDBs should be prescribed in limited cases when indicated (see tailored LA).
- Consent for LA: in the light of Montgomery consent recommendations, all patients should be routinely warned of a risk of nerve injury when routinely undergoing dental local anaesthesia, as already the case in Germany, and in the United Kingdom related to epidural or spinal injections.
- Reduction of epinephrine levels is likely possible for most dental procedures also improving patient safety and minimising systemic effects and reducing problems in medically compromised patients.
- Revalidation of the required cartridge volume is necessary and recommendation for the use of 1.8 mL versus 2.2 mL cartridges will improve patient safety.

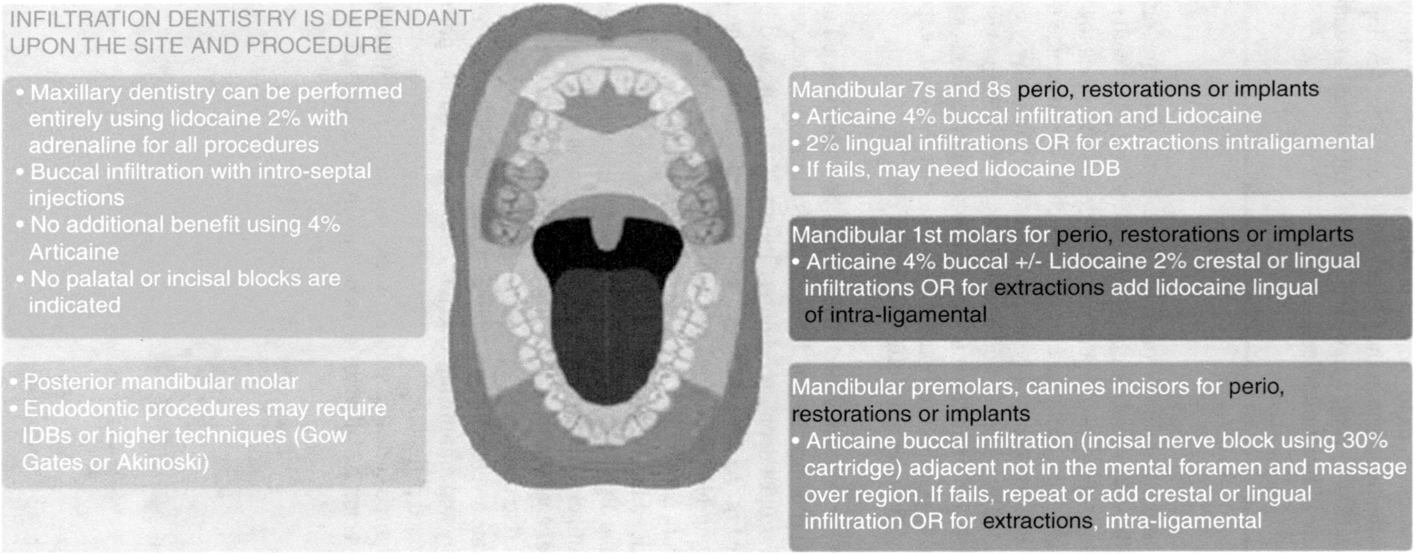

INFILTRATION DENTISTRY IS DEPENDANT UPON THE SITE AND PROCEDURE

- Maxillary dentistry can be performed entirely using lidocaine 2% with adrenaline for all procedures
- Buccal infiltration with intro-septal injections
- No additional benefit using 4% Articaine
- No palatal or incisal blocks are indicated

- Posterior mandibular molar
- Endodontic procedures may require IDBs or higher techniques (Gow Gates or Akinoski)

Mandibular 7s and 8s perio, restorations or implants
- Articaine 4% buccal infiltration and Lidocaine 2% lingual infiltrations OR for extractions intraligamental
- If fails, may need lidocaine IDB

Mandibular 1st molars for perio, restorations or implarts
- Articaine 4% buccal +/- Lidocaine 2% crestal or lingual infiltrations OR for extractions add lidocaine lingual of intra-ligamental

Mandibular premolars, canines incisors for perio, restorations or implants
- Articaine buccal infiltration (incisal nerve block using 30% cartridge) adjacent not in the mental foramen and massage over region. If fails, repeat or add crestal or lingual infiltration OR for extractions, intra-ligamental

Fig. 9.1 Summarising mandibular LA infiltration techniques. (Illustration modified from figure courtesy of Andrew Mason, University Dundee)

References

1. de St Georges J. How dentists are judged by patients. Dent Today. 2004;23(8):96–98–9.
2. Renton T. Prevention and management of perisurgical pain. Dental Update. In Press
3. International Association for the study of pain [IAsp]. 1994. Available from: http://www.iasp-pain.org/AM/Template.cfm?section=pain_Defi.
4. Woolf CJ. What is this thing called pain? J Clin Invest. 2010;120(11):3742–4.
5. Tracey I, et al. Getting the pain you expect: mechanisms of placebo, nocebo and reappraisal effects in humans. Nat Med. 2010;16:1277–83.
6. Kalenderian E, Obadan-Udoh E, Maramaldi P, Etolue J, Yansane A, Stewart D, White J, Vaderhobli R, Kent K, Hebballi NB, Delattre V, Kahn M, Tokede O, Ramoni RB, Walji MF. Classifying adverse events in the dental office. J Patient Saf. 2017; https://doi.org/10.1097/pTs.0000000000000407. Epub ahead of print.
7. Maramaldi P, Walji MF, White J, Etolue J, Kahn M, Vaderhobli R, Kwatra J, Delattre VF, Hebballi NB, Stewart D, Kent K, Yansane A, Ramoni RB, Kalenderian E. How dental team members describe adverse events. J Am Dent Assoc. 2016;147(10):803–11. https://doi.org/10.1016/j.adaj.2016.04.015. Epub 2016 Jun 3.
8. Hiivala N, Mussalo-Rauhamaa H, Tefke HL, Murtomaa H. An analysis of dental patient safety incidents in a patient complaint and healthcare supervisory database in Finland. Acta Odontol scand. 2016;74(2):81–9. https://doi.org/10.3109/00016357.2015.1042040. Epub 2015 May 13.
9. Locker D, Shapiro D, Liddell A. Negative dental experiences and their relationship to dental anxiety. Commun Dent Health. 1996;63(1):86–92.
10. Maggirias J, Locker D. Psychological factors and perceptions of pain associated with dental treatment. Community Dent Oral Epidemiol. 2002;30(2):151–9.
11. Malamed SF. Handbook of Local Anesthesia. 7th Edition: Elsevier Paperback ISBN: 9780323582070; eBook ISBN: 9780323582094.
12. Harris SC. Aspiration before injection of dental local anaesthetics. J Oral Surg. 1957;15:299–303.
13. Shojaei AR, Haas DA. Local anesthetic cartridges and latex allergy: a literature review. J Can Dent Assoc. 2002;68(10):622–6.
14. Syed M, Chopra R, Sachdev V. Allergic reactions to dental materials-a systematic review. J Clin Diagn Res. 2015;9(10):ZE04–9.
15. Goodson JM, Moore PA. Life-threatening reactions after pedodontic sedation: an assessment of narcotic, local anesthetic and antiemetic drug interactions. J Am Dent Assoc. 1983;107:239–45.
16. Niwa H, Tanimoto A, Sugimura M, Morimoto Y, Hanamoto H. Cardiovascular effects of epinephrine under sedation with nitrous oxide, propofol, or midazolam. Oral Surg Oral Med Oral Pathol Oral Radiol Endod. 2006;102(6):e1–9. Epub 2006 Sept 25.
17. Guay J. Methemoglobinemia related to local anesthetics: a summary of 242 episodes. Anesth Analg. 2009;108(3):837–45. https://doi.org/10.1213/ane.0b013e318187c4b1.
18. Botti M, Bucknall T, Manias E. The problem of postoperative pain: issues for future research. Int J Nurs Pract. 2004;10(6):257–63.
19. https://www.aae.org/uploadedfiles/publications_and_research/endodontics_colleagues_for_excellence_newsletter/winter09ecfe.pdf.
20. Vreeland D, Reader A, Beck M, Meyers W, Weaver J. An evaluation of volumes and concentrations of lidocaine in human inferior alveolar nerve block. J Endod. 1989;15:6–12.
21. McLean C, Reader A, Beck M, Meyers WJ. An evaluation of 4% prilocaine and 3% mepivacaine compared to 2% lidocaine (1:100,000 epinephrine) for inferior alveolar nerve block. J Endod. 1993;19:146–50.
22. Hinkley S, Reader A, Beck M, Meyers W. An evaluation of 4% prilocaine with 1:200,000 epinephrine and 2% mepivacaine with levonordefrin compared to 2% lidocaine with 1:100,000 epinephrine for inferior alveolar nerve block. Anesth Prog. 1991;38:84–9.

23. Nusstein J, Reader A, Beck M. Anesthetic efficacy of different volumes of lidocaine with epinephrine for inferior alveolar nerve blocks. Gen Dent. 2002;50:372–5.
24. Mikesell P, Nusstein J, Reader A, Beck M, Weaver J. A comparison of articaine and lidocaine for inferior alveolar nerve blocks. J Endod. 2005;31:265–70.
25. Agren E, Danielsson K. Conduction block analgesia in the mandible. Swed Dent J. 1981;5:81–9.
26. Claffey E, Reader A, Nusstein J, Beck M, Weaver J. Anesthetic efficacy of articaine for inferior alveolar nerve blocks in patients with irreversible pulpitis. J Endod. 2004;30:568–71.
27. Fernandez C, Reader A, Beck M, Nusstein J. A prospective, randomized, double-blind comparison of bupivacaine and lidocaine for inferior alveolar nerve blocks. J Endod. 2005;31:499–503.
28. You TM, Kim K-D, Huh J, Woo E-J, Park W. The influence of mandibular skeletal characteristics on inferior alveolar nerve block anesthesia. J Dent Anesth Pain Med. 2015;15(3):113–9.
29. Kaufman E, Weinstein P, Milgrom P. Difficulties in achieving local anesthesia. J Am Dent Assoc. 1984;108:205–8.
30. Kanaa MD, Meechan JG, Corbett IP, Whitworth JM. Speed of injection influences efficacy of inferior alveolar nerve blocks: a doubleblind randomized controlled trial in volunteers. J Endod. 2006;32:919–23.
31. Meechan JG. The use of the mandibular infiltration anesthetic technique in adults. J Am Dent Assoc. 2011;142(Suppl 3):19S–24S.
32. Yadav S. Anesthetic success of supplemental infiltration in mandibular molars with irreversible pulpitis: a systematic review. J Conserv Dent. 2015;18(3):182–6.
33. Lai TN, Lin CP, Kok SH. Evaluation of mandibular block using a standardize method. Oral Surg Oral Med Oral pathol Oral Radiol Endod. 2006;102:462–8.
34. Meechan JG. How to overcome failed local anaesthesia. Br Dent J. 1999;186(1):15–20.
35. Wali M, Reader A, Beck M, Meyers V. Anesthetic efficacy of lidocaine and epinephrine in human inferior alveolar nerve blocks. J Endod. 1988;14:193. (abstract).
36. Dagher BF, Yared GM, Machtou P. An evaluation of 2% lidocaine with different concentrations of epinephrine for inferior alveolar nerve blocks. J Endod. 1997;23:178–80.
37. Malamed SF, Gagnon S, Leblanc D. Efficacy of articaine: a new amide local anesthetic. J Am Dent Assoc. 2000;131:635–42.
38. Moore PA, Boynes SG, Hersh EV, DeRossi SS, Sollecito TP, Goodson JM, Leonel JS, Floros C, Peterson C, Hutcheson M. Dental anesthesia using 4% articaine 1:200,000 epinephrine: two clinical trials. J Am Dent Assoc. 2006;137:1572–81.
39. Sierra Rebolledo A, Delgado Molina E, Berini Aytis L, Gay Escoda C. Comparative study of the anesthetic efficacy of 4% articaine versus 2% lidocaine in inferior alveolar nerve block during surgical extraction of impacted lower third molars. Med Oral Patol Oral Cir Bucal. 2007;12(2):E139–44.
40. Tortamano IP, Siviero M, Costa CG, Buscariolo IA, Armonia PL. A comparison of the anesthetic efficacy of articaine and lidocaine in patients with irreversible pulpitis. J Endod. 2009;35(2):19166765.
41. Araujo GM, Barbalho JC, Dias TG, Santos Tde S, Vasconcellos RJ, de Morais HH. Comparative analysis between computed and conventional inferior alveolar nerve block techniques. J Craniofac Surg. 2015;26(8):e733–6.
42. Haase A, Reader A, Nusstein J, Beck M, Drum M. Comparing anesthetic efficacy of articaine versus lidocaine as a supplemental buccal infiltration of the mandibular first molar after an inferior alveolar nerve block. J Am Dent Assoc. 2008;139:1228–35.
43. Matthews R, Drum M, Reader A, Nusstein J, Beck M. Articaine for supplemental, buccal mandibular infiltration anesthesia in patients with irreversible pulpitis. J Endod. 2009;35(3):343–6.
44. Kanaa MD, Whitworth JM, Meechan JG. A prospective randomized trial of different supplementary local anesthetic techniques after failure of inferior alveolar nerve block in patients with irreversible pulpitis in mandibular teeth. J Endod. 2012;38(4):421–5. https://doi.org/10.1016/j.joen.2011.12.006. Epub 2012 Feb 2.

45. Dumbrigue HB, Lim MV, Rudman RA, Serraon A. A comparative study of anesthetic techniques for mandibular dental extraction. Am J Dent. 1997;10(6):275–8.
46. Shabazfar N, Daubländer M, Al Nawas B, Kämmerer PW. Periodontal intraligament injection as alternative to inferior alveolar nerve block - metaanalysis of the literature from 1979 to 2012. Clin Oral Investig. 2014;18(2):351–8.
47. Dunbar D, Reader A, Nist R, Beck M, Meyers W. Anesthetic efficacy of the intraosseous injection after an inferior alveolar nerve block. J Endod. 1996;22:481–6.
48. Guglielmo A, Reader A, Nist R, Beck M, Weaver J. Anesthetic efficacy and heart rate effects of the supplemental intraosseous injection of 2% mepivacaine with 1:20,000 levonordefrin. Oral Surg Oral Med Oral Pathol Oral Radiol Endod. 1999;87:284–93.
49. Li C, Yang X, Ma X, Li L, Shi Z. Preoperative oral nonsteroidal anti-inflammatory drugs for the success of the inferior alveolar nerve block in irreversible pulpitis treatment: a systematic review and meta-analysis based on randomized controlled trials. Quintessence Int. 2012;43(3):209–19.
50. Renton T, Adey-Viscuso D, Meechan JG, Yilmaz Z. Trigeminal nerve injuries in relation to the local anaesthesia in mandibular injections. Br Dent J. 2010;209(9):E15.
51. Lima JL Jr, Dias-Ribeiro E, Ferreira-Rocha J, Soares R, Costa FW, Fan S, Sant'ana E. Prospective, double-blind, controlled clinical trial involved 30 patients between the ages of 15 and 46 years who desired extraction of a partially impacted upper third molar with pericoronitis. Anesth Prog. 2013;60(2):42–5.
52. Webber B, Orlansky H, Lipton C, Stevens M. Complications of an intra-arterial injection from an inferior alveolar nerve block. J Am Dent Assoc. 2001;132(12):1702–4.
53. Tzermpos FH, Cocos A, Kleftogiannis M, Zarakas M, Iatrou I. Transient delayed facial nerve palsy after inferior alveolar nerve block anesthesia. Anesth Prog. 2012;59(1):22–7.
54. Cummings DR, Yamashita DD, McAndrews JP. Complications of local anesthesia used in oral and maxillofacial surgery. Oral Maxillofac Surg Clin North Am. 2011;23(3):369–77. https://doi.org/10.1016/j.coms.2011.04.009. Review.
55. Catelani C, Valente A, Rossi A, Bertolai R. Broken anesthetic needle in the pterygomandibular space. Four case reports. Minerva Stomatol. 2013;62(11–12):455–63.
56. von Arx T, Lozanoff S, Zinkernagel M. Ophthalmologic complications after intraoral local anesthesia. Swiss Dent J. 2014;124(7–8):784–806.
57. Baldi C, Bettinelli S, Grossi P, Fausto A, Sardanelli F, Cavalloro F, Allegri M, Braschi A. Ultrasound guidance for locoregional anesthesia: a review. Minerva Anestesiol. 2007;73(11):587–93.
58. Evans G, Nusstein J, Drum M, Reader A, Beck M. A prospective, randomized, double-blind comparison of articaine and lidocaine for maxillary infiltrations. J Endod. 2008;34(4):389–93. https://doi.org/10.1016/j.joen.2008.01.004. Epub 2008 Feb 7.
59. Garisto GA, Gaffen AS, Lawrence HP, Tenenbaum HC, Haas DA. Occurrence of paresthesia after dental local anesthetic administration in the United States. J Am Dent Assoc. 2010;141(7):836–44. Erratum in: J Am Dent Assoc. 2010;141(8):944.
60. Orr DL, Curtis WJ. Oral and maxillofacial surgery, anesthesiology for dentistry, University of Nevada School of Medicine, Las Vegas 89102-2287, USA. J Am Dent Assoc (1939). 2005;136(11):1568–71.
61. National Royal College of Anaesthetists Audit; 2012.
62. Pogrel MA, Thamby S. Permanent nerve involvement resulting from inferior alveolar nerve blocks. J Am Dent Assoc. 2000;131(7):901–7. Erratum in: J Am Dent Assoc 2000 Oct;131(10):1418.
63. Meyers WJ. The use of ultrasound for guiding needle placement for inferior alveolar nerve blocks. Oral Surg Oral Med Oral Pathol Oral Radiol Endod. 1999;87:658–65.
64. Neal JM. Ultrasound-guided regional anesthesia and patient safety: update of an evidence-based analysis. Reg Anesth Pain Med. 2016;41(2):195–204.
65. Hillerup S, Jensen R. Nerve injury caused by mandibular block analgesia. Int J Oral Maxillofac Surg. 2006;35(5):437–43. Epub 2005 Dec 15.
66. Haas DA, Lennon D. A 21 year retrospective study of reports of paresthesia following local anesthetic administration. J Can Dent Assoc. 1995;61(4):319–20, 323–6, 329–30.

67. Haas DA. Articaine and paresthesia: epidemiological studies. J Am Coll Dent. 2006;73(3):5–10. Review.
68. Hillerup S, Jensen RH, Ersboll BK. Trigeminal nerve injury associated with injection of local anesthetics: needle lesion or neurotoxicity? J Am Dent Assoc. 2011;142(5):531–9.
69. Pogrel MA. Permanent nerve damage from inferior alveolar nerve blocks: a current update. J Calif Dent Assoc. 2012;40(10):795–7.
70. Gaffen AS, Haas DA. Retrospective review of voluntary reports of nonsurgical paresthesia in dentistry. J Can Dent Assoc. 2009;75(8):579.
71. Kingon A, Sambrook P, Goss A. Higher concentration local anaesthetics causing prolonged anaesthesia. Do they? A literature review and case reports. Aust Dent J. 2011;56(4):348–51. https://doi.org/10.1111/j.1834-7819.2011.01358.x. Epub 2011 Oct 3. Review.
72. Oliveira PC, Volpato MC, Ramacciato JC, Ranali J. Articaine and lignocaine efficiency in infiltration anaesthesia: a pilot study. Br Dent J. 2004;197(1):45–6; discussion 33.
73. Vähätalo K, Antila H, Lehtinen R. Articaine and lidocaine for maxillary infiltration anesthesia. Anesth Prog. 1993;40(4):114–6.
74. Srinivasan N, Kavitha M, Loganathan CS, Padmini G. Comparison of anesthetic efficacy of 4% articaine and 2% lidocaine for maxillary buccal infiltration in patients with irreversible pulpitis. Oral Surg Oral Med Oral Pathol Oral Radiol Endod. 2009;107:133–6.
75. Lima JL Jr, Dias-Ribeiro E, Ferreira-Rocha J, Soares R, Costa FWG, Fan S, Sant'ana E. Comparison of buccal infiltration of 4% articaine with 1:100,000 and 1:200,000 epinephrine for extraction of maxillary third molars with pericoronitis: a pilot study. Anesth Prog. 2013;60(2):42–5. https://doi.org/10.2344/0003-3006-60.2.42.
76. Bartlett G, Mansoor J. Articaine buccal infiltration vs lidocaine inferior dental block - a review of the literature. Br Dent J. 2016;220(3):117–20. https://doi.org/10.1038/sj.bdj.2016.93.
77. Peters MC, Botero TM. In patients with symptomatic irreversible pulpitis, articaine is 3.6 times more efficacious than lidocaine in achieving anesthetic success when used for supplementary infiltration after mandibular block anesthesia. J Evid Based Dent Pract. 2017;17(2):99–101.
78. Malamed SF. Techniques of maxillary anaesthesia. In: Malamed SF, editor. Handbook of local anaesthesia. 6th ed. St Louis: Mosby Elsevier; 2013. p. 223.
79. Shabazfar N, Daubländer M, Al-Nawas B, Kämmerer PW. Periodonta intraligament injection as alternative to inferior alveolar nerve block - meta-analysis of the literature from 1979 to 2012. Clin Oral Investig. 2014;18(2):351–8.
80. Kämmerer PW, Palarie V, Schiegnitz E, Ziebart T, Al-Nawas B, Daubländer M. Clinical and histological comparison of pulp anesthesia and local diffusion after periodontal ligament injection and intrapapillary infiltration anaesthesia. J Pain Relief. 2012;1:108. https://doi.org/10.4172/2167-0846.1000108-0846.1000108.
81. Zain M, et al. Comparison of anaesthetic efficacy of 4% articaine primary buccal infiltration versus 2% lidocaine inferior alveolar nerve block in symptomatic mandibular first molar teeth. Adults. J Coll Physicians Surg Pak. 2016;26(1):4–8.
82. Poorni S, et al. Anesthetic efficacy of four percent articaine for pulpal anesthesia by using inferior alveolar nerve block and buccal infiltration techniques in patients with pulpitis: a prospective randomized doubleblind clinical trial. J Endod. 2011;37(12):1603–7.
83. Thakare A, Bhate K, Kathariya R. Comparison of 4% articaine and 0.5% bupivacaine anesthetic efficacy in orthodontic extractions: prospective, randomized crossover study. Acta Anaesthesiol Taiwanica. 2014;52(2):59–63.
84. Sanchez-Siles M, Camacho-Alonso F, Salazar-Sanchez N, Aguinaga-Ontoso E, Munoz JG, Calvo-Guirado JL. A low dose of subperiosteal anaesthesia injection versus a high dose of infiltration anaesthesia to minimise the risk of nerve damage at implant placement: a randomised controlled trial. Eur J Oral Implantol. 2016;9(1):59–66.
85. Smith T, Urquiola R, Oueis H, Stenger J. Comparison of articaine and lidocaine in the pediatric population. J Mich Dent Assoc. 2014;96(1):34–7.

86. Arrow P. A comparison of articaine 4% and lignocaine 2% in block and infiltration analgesia in children. Aust Dent J. 2012;57(3):325–33.
87. Kämmerer PW, Schiegnitz E, von Haussen T, Shabazfar N, Kämmerer P, Willershausen B, Al-Nawas B, Daubländer M. Clinical efficacy of a computerised device (STA™) and a pressure syringe (VarioJect INTRA™) for intraligamentary anaesthesia. Eur J Dent Educ. 2015;19(1):16–22.
88. Yapp KE, Hopcraft MS, Parashos P. Articaine: a review of the literature. Br Dental J. 2011;210:323–9.
89. Vree TB, Gielen MJ. Clinical pharmacology and the use of articaine for local and regional anaesthesia. Best Pract Res Clin Anaesthesiol. 2005;19:293–308.
90. Abdulwahab M, Boynes S, Moore P, Seifikar S, Al-Jazzaf A, Alshuraidah A, Zovko J, Close J. The efficacy of six local anesthetic formulations used for posterior mandibular buccal infiltration anesthesia. J Am Dent Assoc. 2009;140(8):1018–24.
91. Becker DE, Reed KL. Essentials of local anesthetic pharmacology. Anesth Prog. 2006;53:98–109.
92. Kämmerer PW, Schneider D, Palarie V, Schiegnitz E, Daubländer M. Comparison of anesthetic efficacy of 2 and 4% articaine in inferior alveolar nerve block for tooth extraction-a double-blinded randomized clinical trial. Clin Oral Investig. 2017;21(1):397–403.
93. Senes AM, Calvo AM, Colombini-Ishikiriama BL, Goncalves PZ, Dionísio TJ, Sant'ana E, Brozoski DT, Lauris JR, Faria FA, Santos CF. Efficacy and safety of 2% and 4% articaine for lower third molar surgery. J Dent Res. 2015;94(9 Suppl):166s–73s. https://doi.org/10.1177/0022034515596313. Epub 2015 Jul 22.
94. Zurfluh MA, Daubländer M, van Waes HJ. Comparison of two epinephrine concentrations in an articaine solution for local anesthesia in children. Swiss Dent J. 2015;125(6):698–709.
95. Malamed S. 1.8 or 2.2 ml? How much anaesthetic is enough? Personal communication.
96. Shahidi Bonjar AH. Syringe micro vibrator (SMV) a new device being introduced in dentistry to alleviate pain and anxiety of intraoral injections, and a comparative study with a similar device. Ann Surg Innov Res. 2011;5:1–5.
97. Katyal V. The efficacy and safety of articaine versus lignocaine in dental treatments: a meta-analysis. J Dent. 2010;38:307–17.
98. Brandt RG, Anderson PF, McDonald NJ, Sohn W, Peters MC. The pulpal anesthetic efficacy of articaine versus lidocaine in dentistry: a meta-analysis. J Am Dent Assoc. 2011;142(5):493–504.
99. Kung J, McDonagh M, Sedgley CM. Does articaine provide an advantage over lidocaine in patients with symptomatic irreversible pulpitis? A systematic review and meta-analysis. J Endod. 2015;41(11):1784–94.
100. Daublander M, Mauller R, Lipp MD. The incidence of complications associated with local anaesthesia in dentistry. Anesth prog. 1997;44(4):132–41.

Temporomandibular Disorders for the General Dental Practitioner

10

Emma Beecroft, Chris Penlington, Hannah Desai, and Justin Durham

Learning Objectives

- Examination, diagnosis and biopsychosocial management of TMD in primary care.
- The presenting features and common signs and symptoms of TMD.
- Red flag symptoms which mimic TMD and require onward referral.
- Integrated treatment plan.

Temporomandibular disorder (TMD) is a collective term for conditions affecting the temporomandibular joint (TMJ), muscles of mastication (MOM) or both [1, 2]. Temporomandibular disorders (TMDs) can be acute or persistent. Acute TMD usually has a short duration and identifiable precipitating factor, e.g. temporomandibular joint pain and restricted opening following protracted molar root canal treatment. The pain felt is protective, allowing reparation of damage [3].

Approximately 10% of all TMD cases progress to a persistent (or chronic) condition [4]. Persistent TMD involves protracted pain (>3 months), which no longer serves any reparative function [3]. Persistent TMDs demonstrate increased pain intensity compared to acute TMDs [5], with a quarter of cases demonstrating functional disability [2]. Persistent TMDs demonstrate significant biopsychosocial consequences [3], impacting on patients' work and home environment, affecting social engagement and personal relationships [2, 6, 7].

E. Beecroft · C. Penlington · H. Desai · J. Durham (✉)
School of Dental Sciences, Newcastle University, Newcastle upon Tyne, UK
e-mail: emma.beecroft@newcastle.ac.uk; Chris.Penlington@newcastle.ac.uk; Hannah.Desai@newcastle.ac.uk; Justin.durham@newcastle.ac.uk

10.1   Epidemiology

TMDs are the most common cause of chronic pain in the orofacial region [1]. Prevalence in the general population is reported at 10–15% [8]. Incidence of TMDs are marginally higher in females compared to males, however, females have substantially increased odds of generating persistent TMD [5]. TMD presentation follows an inverted "U" trend, with the peak incidence being between 18 and 44 years old [3, 4, 6]. Interestingly, unlike most chronic pain conditions, there appears to be no causal association between socioeconomic group and incidence of TMD [3, 5, 6].

10.2   Presenting Features

Mild to moderate pain intensity and disability are the most commonly reported presenting features [5]. Around 65% of patients report recurrent pain with their TMD, demonstrating classic cycles of remission and flare-up [5]. A single episode of pain is reported in 12% of cases, whilst 19% report persistent pain [5].

Practitioners must be aware of the propensity for referred pain in the head and neck region [9]; the most common sites of referred pain from palpation of facial musculature are shown in Fig. 10.1. Awareness that TMD pain can present in areas distant from those expected, and conversely, examination of muscles of mastication can trigger pain in distant sites, is essential so as not to misdiagnose.

With regards to the temporomandibular joint itself, jaw stiffness, reduced mobility and masticatory difficulty are common presenting features, with 41% of TMD cases demonstrating restricted opening [2]. Joint noises can also be present, which may or may not cause pain [2].

10.3   Aetiology

TMDs have a complex multifactorial aetiology with no singular "cause". A number of biopsychosocial factors play a role in initiating, predisposing and perpetuating TMDs and their roles are still not fully understood [10]. The genotype of an individual helps determine their biological susceptibility to TMD, whilst psychological and behavioural factors influence the pain experience [6]. Other factors implicated include, but are not limited to joint and muscle trauma; parafunction; and sensitisation of peripheral and central pain processing pathways [4, 6]. One factor historically associated with the aetiology of TMDs has now been shown not to play a role: orthodontic treatment neither causes nor treats TMD [2, 6, 11].

10.4   The Influence of Comorbidities

There are a number of comorbidities that, when present, increase the propensity towards symptomatic persistent TMD with a consequentially poorer prognostic outcome. Early recognition of susceptible patients is essential to provide targeted early

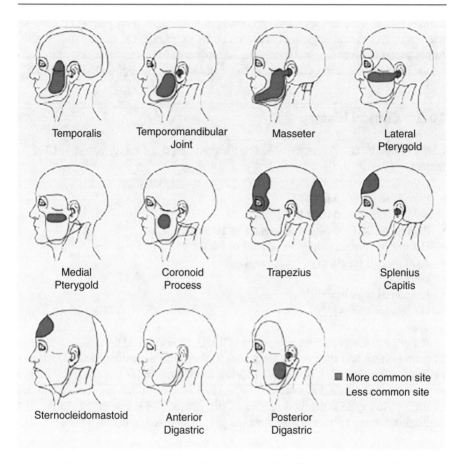

Fig. 10.1 Map of referred pain generated by palpation of labelled anatomic areas. With permissions from [9]

intervention in a bid to control symptoms before neuroplastic changes occur that result in central sensitisation.

For some patients, painful TMD may be a single symptom of a systemic condition (e.g. rheumatoid arthritis, fibromyalgia), in such cases management should be completed in conjunction with physicians responsible for the patient's systemic well-being [3]. For others, comorbid presentation of TMD with pain conditions in other areas of the body (e.g. chronic back pain) indicates potential dysregulation of pain regulatory pathways [2, 4, 6], generating hyperalgesia and diffuse allodynia through sensitisation of the peripheral and/or central nervous system described as "pain amplification" [4, 6]. Referral to a general medical practitioner (GMP) should be considered for patients presenting with undiagnosed widespread body pain.

Psychological factors such as anxiety, depression and catastrophising thoughts have been shown to be significant risk factors for both the development of painful TMDs and the transition from acute to persistent pain states [6, 12]. Cognitive, emotional and behavioural factors associated with psychological conditions will influence how a patient reacts to, processes and manages their pain [11]. Patients who recognise that their pain is exacerbated by psychological factors may benefit from specialist psychological treatment. In most areas, this can be accessed by self-referral to the local improving Access to Psychological Therapies (IAPT) service.

10.5 Clinical History

GDPs should be competent to recognise the common signs and symptoms of TMDs including [3, 10]:

- Pain in and around the TMJ
- Pain in and around the MOM
- Pain in the TMJ or MOM worsened by function
- History of pain on palpation of TMJ or MOM
- Joint sounds (click, pop, snap, crepitus)
- Headaches
- Restricted joint mobility
- Otalgia [±tinnitus]

If signs and symptoms are suggestive of TMD, GDPs should first rule out the pain of dental origin and then refine their pain history with a specific TMD focus. For patients with otalgia with or without tinnitus, a GMP referral is warranted for further assessment. The medical mnemonic SOCRATES is an extremely useful tool that can be utilised to create a detailed picture of the patient's pain complaint. Table 10.1 highlights potential findings from detailed pain history suggestive of TMD.

Table 10.1 Example pain history for TMD case utilising socrates mnemonic

Site	Primarily affected: TMJ, MOM, Ear Consider referral pathways for pain (Fig. 10.1)
Onset	Acute TMD: usually has identifiable precipitating event Chronic TMD: more difficult to pinpoint Could be sudden or gradual Link to dental treatment or trauma
Character	Dull, deep, aching, throbbing Usually continuous ± acute exacerbations Cyclical nature: periods of flare-up and remission
Radiation and referral (see Fig. 10.1)	Most common referral patterns: ear, angle of jaw, temple, teeth
Association and alleviating factors	Rest/analgesics may improve Function may worsen
Timing—duration and frequency	How long in total has the pain been present: Short duration in acute TMD, Long history for persistent TMDs Most likely to present continuously Diurnal variation pattern sometimes seen (worse in the morning, eases through the day or vice versa) Duration of pain can be a prognostic indicator
Exacerbating factors	Chewing/talking/yawning/movement
Severity. Pain score out of 10 with 10 being "the worst pain imaginable"	Variable

Adapted from Durham et al. [3]

Specific questioning with regards to headache profile is recommended as headaches can form a component of the TMD or could be part of a mimicking or comorbid condition e.g. temporal arteritis, or migraine.

10.6 Clinical Examination

It is assumed that a minimal expected standard from every clinical contact would include visual extra-oral examination of the patient's face and neck, palpation to assess any lymphadenopathy, examination of intraoral soft tissues to rule out soft tissue lesions and dental examination to exclude frank dental or periodontal pathology. For suspected TMD further examination should include assessment of cranial nerves (at least the facial and trigeminal nerves). Clear concise guidance on how to complete cranial nerve tests can be found at https://geekymedics.com/cranial-nerve-exam/ [13].

In patients suspected of TMD, TMJ and MOM should be examined for familiar pain. Familiar pain is pain precipitated during the examination that is representative of the patient's normal pain experience [11]. Ensuring a "familiar" nature of pain with clinical examination equates to a clinically meaningful result, ruling out false positives and incidental findings [12].

10.7 TMJ Examination

International recommendations advise palpation of the TMJ over its lateral pole [12], through the mandibular opening, closing, protrusion and lateral excursions. An alternative or adjunct to this would be intra-aural palpation of the joint in the external auditory meatus. The mandibular motions should be repeated three times; a "familiar" response to one-third of the cycles represents a positive finding [12]. Deviation along the arc of mandibular opening, measured maximal inter incisal opening (unassisted and assisted) in millimetres and protrusive and lateral excursive range of opening should all be documented as they can give indicators towards specific diagnoses (see Sect. 10.12).

Presentation of joint noises can be sporadic and clinical detection of TMJ noises is difficult [12]. Due to this, joint noises can be documented as positive during the clinical examination if the patient self-reports hearing joint noise(s) in the last 30 days and/or noise is heard by the patient or clinician during the examination [12]. Another consideration would be the use of a stethoscope to auscultate for faint noises that are not palpable.

10.8 Muscles of Mastication

All accessible aspects of both temporalis and masseter should be palpated bimanually (where possible) from superior to inferior attachments. Palpation of temporalis and masseter muscles alone has been shown to provide diagnostic validity [12].

Documentation of "familiar" pain on palpation, location of pain, radiation of pain and presence of trigger point should be summarised. Palpation of additional musculature e.g. lateral pterygoid, medial pterygoid, digastric, etc. is only required when clinically indicated for instance when the pain or dysfunction is reported in the anatomical boundaries or movements associated with these muscles [12].

10.9   Biopsychosocial Evaluation

Physical clinical examination alone is no longer considered an adequate assessment for TMD in isolation. It is widely recognised that the way an individual feels pain is influenced by cognitive, emotional and behavioural factors [12], which physical examination would fail to recognise. Psychosocial comorbidity has been shown to have an impact on pain severity and development of persistent pain and affects both prognosis and treatment outcome [10, 12].

Assessment of pain intensity and emotional functioning should cover behavioural assessment (how the patient and their friends and family respond to their pain), the patient's beliefs, attitudes and expectations in addition to their mood (e.g. anxiety and depression). In the related area of back pain, a brief screening instrument has been shown to be successful in allocating patients to appropriate treatment [14]. By taking into account relevant psychosocial factors including fear of pain, low mood (depression), avoidance of functional activity and thinking the worst (catastrophising), patients are treated according to stratified risk [14]. Similar psychosocial risk factors have been reported for TMDs [15], therefore, an adapted version of this instrument may also be helpful in this population. The acronym FLATS shown in Fig. 10.2 can be utilised as a brief psychosocial screening tool. A positive

Agreement with one or more items below, suggests medium risk and the need for more frequent appointments for monitoring, support and reinforcement of self-care recommendations.

Agreement with three or more, suggests high risk and consideration of referral to specialist services.

Fear of Pain	Do you worry that you could cause injury by biting, chewing or making certain movements?
Low mood	In general, have you been enjoying the things you used to enjoy?
Avoidance	Do you avoid doing things in case of making your pain worse?
Thinking the Worst	Do you have thoughts liks 'it's terrible and it's never going to get any better?'
Social Impact	Does your pain have an impact on other people?

Fig. 10.2   FLATS mnemonic: a brief screening and triage tool of psychosocial risk factors in TMD

response to one or more of the items flags the need for more frequent appointments for monitoring, support and reinforcement of self-care advice with the GDP. In some cases, self-referral to local IAPT services may also be appropriate, as previously discussed. For patients who show three or more of the risk factors, referral to a specialist service if available, or liaison with the patient's GP about referral to specialist pain management services, is advised.

If time allows, a more comprehensive biopsychosocial (so-called "Axis II") assessment is covered in the diagnostic criteria for temporomandibular disorders (DC/TMD) with psychosocial screening questionnaires available to print and utilise at https://ubwp.buffalo.edu/rdc-tmdinternational/tmd-assessmentdiagnosis/dc-tmd/ [16]. Depending on patients' responses, referral for a more comprehensive psychological evaluation and adjunctive psychological intervention through the patient's GMP may be appropriate [3, 10].

10.10 Red Flags

A small number of dangerous conditions exist that can produce signs and symptoms which mimic TMDs. Positive findings of "red flag" signs and symptoms in either history or examination must be appropriately investigated with prompt referral to secondary care setting or appropriate medical specialties. Table 10.2 highlights red flag features.

10.11 Imaging

Imaging of TMJ for TMD diagnosis is a contentious issue for two main reasons. The first is that a high proportion of asymptomatic individuals can show "positive" findings, on plain film, cone-beam CT and MRI [17–19]. The second is that, regardless of findings, management strategies and treatment decisions are rarely affected. This makes the associated radiation dose (plain film radiographs/CBCT/CT) critical to justify.

Imaging should be provided only if a clear clinical justification is present, and therefore routine imaging for screening of TMD is inappropriate.

10.12 Diagnosis

Diagnosis provides legitimacy for those experiencing TMD and is the foundation for improved self-perception, increased understanding and provision of coping strategies [7]. Diagnosis should ideally be delivered at the first point of contact, as research has shown that a lack of diagnosis, or a delay in its provision, can cause uncertainty for patients, resulting in negative impacts on the sufferer's condition and their daily lives [7]. By far the most common overall diagnosis on examination is myalgia with arthralgia [5]. A diagnostic guide abstracted and modified from DC/

Table 10.2 Red flag signs and symptoms

Sign	Possible cause
Previous malignancy	Potential for new primary, recurrence or metastases
Lymphadenopathy or neck mass	Neoplastic, infective or autoimmune cause
Jaw claudication (Cramp-like pain in tongue or jaw)	Neoplastic, temporal arteritis
Unplanned weight loss	Neoplastic, systemic illness
Pyrexia	Infective
Neurological signs/symptoms • Acute onset loss of smell • Acute onset loss of hearing • Acute onset visual problems • Paraesthesia • Motor function changes	Neoplastic, infective or autoimmune cause
Pain with exertion, coughing or sneezing (suggests raised intracranial pressure)	Neoplastic or infective cause
Nasal symptoms (persistent and profuse bleeding or (purulent) discharge)	Neoplastic or infective
Acute onset of profound, or worsening, trismus	Neoplastic, infective or traumatic cause
Persistent hoarseness of the voice (>3 weeks)	Neoplastic
Persistent mouth ulcer(s) (>3 weeks)	Neoplastic
Occlusal changes	Neoplastic, traumatic, growth disturbance
Unilateral headache, jaw claudication, flu-like symptoms, vision disturbances, inflammation of temporal artery, trismus in patient age range: >50 years old F > M	Temporal arteritis

TMD [12] which links patient signs, symptoms and clinical examination findings are shown in Table 10.3.

10.13 Management

Long-standing international consensus is that first-line care for patients with TMDs should be reversible and non-invasive [3, 10, 20]. The evidence base for this claim is irrefutable, with data suggesting between 75% and 90% of patients will be responsive to conservative management [21]. The Royal College of Surgeons' Primary Care guidance for TMD explains that the goals of management are:

- Encouragement of self-management of the condition through education.
- Reducing the (impact of) pain associated with the condition.
- Decreasing functional limitation caused by the condition [3].

Table 10.3   Diagnostic guide linking clinical history and examination results to diagnosis

Clinical history	Clinical examination findings	Specific findings related to pain or complaint	Diagnosis
Pain in the Jaw, temple, in the ear or in front of the ear **AND** Pain modified with jaw movement, function or parafunction	Confirmation of pain in temporalis or masseter **AND** "Familiar" pain in masseter or temporalis produced during the examination	The pain of muscular origin	**Myalgia**
		Pain localised to the site of palpation	**Local myalgia**
		Pain spreads beyond the site of palpation but within the boundary of muscle	**Myofascial pain**
		The pain reported at a site beyond the boundary of the muscle being palpated	**Myofascial pain with referral**
Headache of any type in the temple **AND** Headache modified with jaw movement, function or parafunction	"Familiar" headache pain in the temple area produced during examination **AND** Conformation of headache location in the area of the temporalis		**Headache attributed to TMD**
In the last 30 days, any TMJ noise present with jaw movement or function **OR** Patient reports any noise during the exam ± TMJ pain	Clicking, popping ± snapping detected during palpation of 1/3 repetitions of opening/closing, lateral excursion or protrusion	No locking but joint noise	**Disc displacement with reduction**
In the last 30 days, any TMJ noise present with jaw movement or function **OR** Patient reports any noise during the exam **AND** in the last 30 days jaw locks with limited mouth opening even for a moment ± TMJ pain		In the last 30 days jaw locks with limited mouth opening even for a moment then unlocks	**Disc displacement with reduction with intermittent locking**
Jaw locking so mouth would not open all of the ways **AND** Limitation in jaw opening severe enough to limit jaw opening and interfere with the ability to eat	Maximum assisted opening with passive stretch <40 mm The presence of TMJ noise on examination does not exclude this diagnosis		**Disc displacement without reduction with the limited opening "Closed lock"**
	Maximum assisted opening with passive stretch >40 mm The presence of TMJ noise on examination does not exclude this diagnosis		**Disc displacement without reduction without limited opening**

(continued)

Table 10.3 (continued)

Clinical history	Clinical examination findings	Specific findings related to pain or complaint	Diagnosis
In the last 30 days any TMJ noise present with jaw movement or function **OR** Patient reports any noise during the exam ± TMJ pain	Crepitus detected during examination		**Degenerative joint disease**
In the last 30 days jaw locking or catching in a wide-open mouth position, even for a moment, so it could not close from the wide-open position ± TMJ pain	A positive finding of "open lock" which requires manipulation (self or clinician) to reduce	Self-manoeuvre required by the patient to reduce the dislocation	**Subluxation "open lock"**
		Clinician manoeuvre required to reduce the dislocation	**Luxation "open lock"**
Pain in the Jaw, temple, in the ear or in front of the ear **AND** Pain modified with jaw movement, function or parafunction	Confirmation of pain in the area of the TMJ **AND** "Familiar" pain in the TMJ produced during the examination		**Arthralgia**

Adapted from Schiffman et al. [12]

All treatments for TMDs should be delivered within a biopsychosocial framework taking account of biological, psychological and social factors [22, 23]. Psychosocial factors have been shown to be the stronger predictors of outcome in persistent pain [23]. Here we describe the importance of social aspects of care, usual treatment recommendations, psychological and finally biological aspects of management.

10.14 Social Influence of the General Dental Practitioner

Aspects of the interaction between patient and GDP will be crucial to successful patient engagement in self-management, which is arguably the most important part of an intervention. Patients need to feel that their practitioner is listening to them, believing their account and taking their concerns seriously. It is important also that they believe their treatment provider to be competent and knowledgeable to treat their condition. It is worth taking the time to listen carefully and clarify the patient's reports of symptoms and validate their experience since the ability of the patient to engage fully with treatment suggestions will rest on the quality of their relationship with the GDP.

10.15 Education and Reassurance

Time should be spent after the provision of a diagnosis of TMD, to explain this to the patient, discuss its aetiology and provide positive reassurance with regards to its benign and usually non-progressive nature [10, 23]. The power of such reassurance should not be underestimated; delay in the provision of this important step has been shown to subjectively increase anxiety and exacerbate symptom severity [7].

Education at this stage should include a discussion about the role of psychological factors including anxiety, depression and thinking the worst. These do not cause pain but are known to contribute to the intensity and maintenance of pain once it is present, and are likely themselves, to be triggered by pain. For further information about psychological factors in pain, patients can be directed to online resources such as "live well with pain" at my.livewellwithpain.co.uk [24]. it is important at an early stage also to stress the importance of active engagement with self-management strategies and that the outcome of treatment will be related more to what patients do themselves than on treatment received passively. Helpful, free animations are available for patients on "What to do about jaw pain" (https://www.youtube.com/watch ?v=IkpY37aMOMY&list=PL0Zkwya_9eK9dUJbeyARqIxupd8i53EbJ&index=1) and "Self-management in TMD" (https://www.youtube.com/watch?v=dfjdyWoRw Nw&list=PL0Zkwya_9eK9dUJbeyARqIxupd8i53EbJ&index=3).

10.16 Self-Management

Early-stage acute TMD management should include jaw rest and a soft diet in times of acute pain [23]. Parafunctional activities (e.g. nail-biting, jaw clenching/grinding, gum chewing) are likely to contribute to, and also present as a result of TMD pain [2]. Early cessation of such activities can help prevent exacerbation of the condition [23]. Local measures, such as utilising covered ice or moist heat application to affected musculature and facial massage have been shown to provide symptomatic relief and should be encouraged as part of a self-care regime [23].

Poor sleep quality has a reciprocal relationship with chronic pain [25] by lowering pain tolerance leading to pain amplification. Conversely, persistent pain makes both initiation and maintenance of sleep problematic [25]. A helpful leaflet about sleep and pain is available from painconcern.org.uk/sleep [26].

Patients can be directed to simple techniques such as diaphragmatic breathing and sleep hygiene recommendations (see Table 10.4), to utilise at home to improve quality and quantity of sleep, facilitate relaxation and in turn build resilience [10].

10.17 Smoking and Caffeine

Smokers have an increased incidence of TMDs compared to non-smokers. This relationship is more pronounced in younger age groups (18- to 29-year-olds). Sanders et al. found risk of persistent TMD was more than four times as high compared with older adults who had never smoked [27]. There are a number of reasons smoking may affect the incidence of TMDs: nicotine has been shown to modify pain perception, chronic exposure to nicotine is linked to hyperalgesia, and smoking is associated with a worse psychosocial profile (anxiety, depression, perceived stress) [27]. Smoking cessation advice is a simple management strategy that

Table 10.4 Advice for positive sleep hygiene [26]

Routines	Keep to a regular routine, going to bed and getting up at a similar time each day. Before bed spend 20 min winding down in a similar way each night, perhaps including some relaxation exercises. Don't spend long periods of time in bed unable to sleep (unless you feel very relaxed). Get up, move to a different room if possible and do something which is not stimulating. Only return to bed once you feel sleepy.
Environment	Make sure your bedroom is comfortable and uncluttered. Do not watch TV or eat food in bed or use the bed for any other activity that tends to keep you awake in your experience. Keep the temperature and noise distractions low if possible.
Lifestyle	Limit caffeine and alcohol consumption. Do not eat large meals late at night. Make sure you get plenty of exercises, but don't engage in strenuous exercise within an hour or two of going to bed.

supports chronic pain management and systemic health promotion and should be encouraged for all TMD patients.

Excessive caffeine levels have been shown to impact negatively chronic pain conditions [28]. Caffeine stimulates the release of catecholamines e.g. adrenaline, which sensitise muscle nociceptors, increasing the perception of pain [28]. Patients with persistent TMD should be advised to moderate their caffeine intake, switching to decaffeinated alternatives where possible [9, 29].

10.18 Splint Therapy

Splints are usually worn through the night to protect the dentition from parafunction and provide an element of biofeedback to the patient [3]. Splints can be worn on upper or lower arches and there is no evidence for improved efficacy for one over the other [30]. Soft polyethylene material or hard acrylic materials can be used but full coverage of all of the teeth in the arch is advisable to protect against unfavourable over eruption and dentoalveolar compensation [30]. Splints should be monitored by GDPs at routine dental health checks, ensuring positive fit and even occlusal contacts in the intercuspal position when relevant to the type of splint. If excessive wear or damage is present, they should be replaced. Once a patient's TMD has stabilised, continued use of the appliance is not essential, it can however be reintroduced should the patient suffer cyclical flare-up.

10.19 Physiotherapy and Acupuncture

Physiotherapy can reduce muscular discomfort and improve joint function [3]. Evidence confirms short-term symptomatic improvement for TMD cases, but there is no evidence this improvement is consistently maintained [3]. Physiotherapy at the very least provides short-term relief and promotes engagement in self-care regime;

when prescribed appropriately physiotherapy will do no harm and so the consensus is supportive for this form of non-invasive care.

Acupuncture for the care of myogenous TMDs has been shown to reduce pain intensity and a specific improvement in masseteric tenderness has been demonstrated [10]. To arrange physiotherapy and acupuncture for patients, GDPs can liaise with GMPs for onward NHS referral if the service is available in the locality. Alternatively, when the potential benefits of such treatments are explained to patients they may opt to directly access treatment providers through the private sector.

10.20 Psychological Management

As discussed above, all intervention strategies for TMDs are integrated with an understanding of psychological principles. Referral for specialist psychological input is appropriate for patients with high levels of anxiety and depression or whose attempts to engage in self-management appear to be blocked by psychological factors. It is important that patients understand that a referral for psychological therapy is not an indication that professionals believe their pain is psychological or "in their head". Referrals should be discussed and agreed upon with patients before being made, and a clear rationale given. Usually, this will be that it is stressful to live with pain, and this stress is likely to have an impact on symptom maintenance and intensity without careful psychological management. As described previously, patients may opt to self-refer to local IAPT services or to seek a referral from their GMP to specialist pain management services, which include psychology provision within an integrated biopsychosocial framework.

Psychologists may employ a range of different interventions in pain management settings. Of these, cognitive behavioural therapy (CBT) has been reported as successful for TMDs [31]. The therapy supports pain management through patient education and the development of coping strategies, which can result in alteration of the perception of pain [3, 10]. Evidence suggests CBT could provide benefit for most TMD patients, with positive long-term improvement outcomes demonstrated for pain intensity, depression and activity interference [3, 32, 33]. Where indicated, referrals for psychological input should be expedited at an early stage of treatment to facilitate swift intervention [3].

10.21 Pharmacological Management

For any pharmacological management strategy, it is the GDP's responsibility to **check for contraindications and interactions** and to prescribe appropriately on an individual basis. Ensuring patients are fully informed with regards to risks, benefits and potential side effects of the medication are imperative and documentation of these discussions must form part of the patient records.

10.21.1 Simple Analgesics

Systemic nonsteroidal anti-inflammatory drugs (NSAIDs), such as ibuprofen, are widely used for TMD with an inflammatory component, despite little evidence to support their benefit. Topical use of ibuprofen gel may benefit myofascial TMD when applied to the affected musculature. Additional use of paracetamol with NSAIDs may provide sufficient relief to allow a decrease in the NSAID dose, negating potential side effects [3]. Over-the-counter analgesics should be used for short-term acute pain only. Long-term use (>15 days) puts patients at risk of medication overuse headache.

10.21.2 Neuromodulatory Agents

Neuromodulatory agents in the form of antidepressant medications (amitriptyline) or antiepileptic medications (gabapentin) can be used off-licence for persistent pain conditions such as TMDs. Evidence for their effectiveness specifically with regards to TMDs is scant and often empirical [1]. Evidence for the positive response to other chronic pain conditions is often extrapolated to suggest benefits for TMDs [23]. This treatment modality is best left to secondary care through close liaison with the patient's GMP.

10.21.3 Botulinum Toxin

Localised placement of botulinum toxin (BT) blocks the activity of muscles, inhibits the release of inflammatory mediators and alters pain processing pathways, reducing central sensitisation [34]. All of these features suggest BT placement should positively benefit myofascial TMDs but studies have provided equivocal or conflicting results [35–37]. Recent findings in animal studies where BT was delivered to MOM show a reduction in bone volume and hypertrophic bone proliferation in and around TMJ [38]. This finding clearly raises concern about BT's long-term use and further research is required to prove potential benefits outweigh risks of treatment [10].

10.22 Surgical Management

Surgical interventions to manage arthrogenous TMDs include, arthroscopy, arthrocentesis, arthroplasty or joint replacement [23, 39]. A recent systematic review found insufficient evidence to support surgical interventions [8]. As the vast majority of TMDs have been shown to respond to conservative treatments, the morbidity associated with surgical techniques is difficult to justify, provision of such care remains controversial and should be restricted to specific cases with clear indications in centres with the appropriate expertise [39].

10.23   Referral to Secondary Care

In cases where the diagnosis is unclear, or symptoms become chronic or worsen despite initial management, then secondary care referral should be made. Additional support may also be required for patients with marked psychological distress, hypervigilance of symptoms and complex widespread pain [23].

10.24   Conclusion

TMDs present commonly in general dental practice. GDPs role lies in: early diagnosis, effective education and reassurance, appropriate initial management and sensible follow-up. The multifactorial nature of TMDs and wide diagnostic remit makes a detailed history and examination essential to provide appropriate management of both physical symptoms and concomitant psychosocial elements. A biopsychosocial approach should be adopted for TMD patients, with biological, psychological and social elements of management being delivered through a single integrated treatment plan.

When primary care efforts have been exhausted or for other previously outlined reasons, referral to secondary care services does not negate primary care's role in continuing to implement, reinforce and monitor conservative management techniques which are within their remit. Where indicated, secondary care intervention should be completed in conjunction with primary care management strategies to provide the best prognostic opportunity for patients.

References

1. Durham J, Wassell RW. Recent advancements in temporomandibular disorders (TMDs). Rev Pain. 2011;5(1):18–25.
2. Ohrbach R, Fillingim RB, Mulkey F, Gonzalez Y, Gordon S, Gremillion H, Lim PF, Ribeiro-Dasilva M, Greenspan JD, Knott C, Maixner W, Slade G. Clinical findings and pain symptoms as potential risk factors for chronic TMD: descriptive data and empirically identified domains from the OPPERA case control study. J Pain. 2011;12(11):T27–45.
3. Durham J, Aggarwal VA, Davies SJ, Harrison SD, Jagger RG, Leeson R, et al. Temporomandibular Disorders (TMDs): an update and management guidance for primary care from the UK Specialist interest Group in Orofacial Pain and TMDs (USOT). 2013. www. rcseng.ac.uk/fds/publications-clinical-guidelines/clinical_guidelines.
4. Bonato LL, Quinelato V, De Felipe Cordeiro PC, De Sousa EB, Tesch R, Casado PL. Association between temporomandibular disorders and pain in other regions of the body. J Oral Rehabil. 2017;44:9–12.
5. Slade GD, Bair E, Greenspan JD, Dubner R, Fillingim RB, Diatchenko L, et al. Signs and symptoms of first-onset TMD and sociodemographic predictors of its development: the OPPERA prospective cohort study. J Pain. 2013;14(12):T20–32.
6. Maixner W, Diatchenko L, Dubner R, Fillingim RB, Greenspan JD, Knott C, Ohrbach R, Weir B, Slade GD. Orofacial pain prospective evaluation and risk assessment study-the OPPERA study. J Pain. 2011;12(11):T4–11.

7. Durham J, Steele JG, Wassell RW, Exley C. Living with uncertainty: temporomandibular disorders. J Dent Res. 2010;89:827–30.
8. List T, Axelsson S. Management of TMD: evidence from systematic reviews and metaanalyses. J Oral Rehabil. 2010;37(6):430–51.
9. Wright EF. Referred craniofacial pain patterns in patients with temporomandibular disorder. J Am Dent Assoc. 2000;131(9):1307–15. https://doi.org/10.14219/jada.archive.2000.0384.
10. Durham J, Newton-John TRO, Zakrzewska JM. Clinical review: Temporomandibular disorders. BMJ. 2015;350:h1154.
11. Luther F, Layton S, McDonald F. Orthodontics for treating temporomandibular joint (TMJ) disorders. Cochrane Database Syst Review. 2010;7:CD006541.
12. Schiffman E, Ohrbach R, Truelove E, Look J, Anderson G, Goulet JP, et al. Diagnostic Criteria for Temporomandibular Disorders (DC/TMD) for clinical and research applications: recommendations of the international RDC/TMD Consortium Network and Orofacial Pain Special Interest Group. J Oral Facial Pain Headache. 2014;28:6–27.
13. Bargiela D. (2018) Cranial nerve exam-OSCE guide. Available from: https://geekymedics.com/cranial-nerve-exam/. Accessed 1 Nov 2018.
14. Hill JC, Whitehurst DG, Lewis M, Bryan S, Dunn KM, Foster NE, Konstantinou K, Main CJ, Mason E, Somerville S, Sowden G. Comparison of stratified primary care management for low back pain with current best practice (STarT Back): a randomised controlled trial. Lancet. 2011;378(9802):1560–71.
15. Velly AM, Look JO, Carlson C, Lenton PA, Kang W, Holcroft CA, Fricton JR. The effect of catastrophizing and depression on chronic pain–a prospective cohort study of temporomandibular muscle and joint pain disorders. Pain. 2011;152(10):2377–83.
16. International Network for Orofacial Pain and Related Disorders Methodology (INFORM). Available from: https://ubwp.buffalo.edu/rdc-tmdinternational/tmd-assessmentdiagnosis/dc-tmd/. Accessed 1 Nov 2018.
17. Larheim TA, Westesson P, Sano T. Temporomandibular joint disk displacement: comparison in asymptomatic volunteers and patients. Radiology. 2001;218(2):428–32.
18. Larheim TA, Katzberg RW, Westesson PL, Tallents RH, Moss ME. MR evidence of temporomandibular joint fluid and condyle marrow alterations: occurrence in asymptomatic volunteers and symptomatic patients international. J Oral Maxillofac Surg. 2001;30(2):113–7.
19. Bakke M, Peterson A, Wiese M. Bony deviations revealed by cone beam computed tomography of the temporomandibular joint in subjects without ongoing pain. J Oral Facial Pain Headache. 2014;28:331–7.
20. Albino J. Management of temporomandibular disorders. National institutes of health technology assessment conference statement. JADA. 1996;127:1595–606.
21. Greene CS. The etiology of temporomandibular disorders: implications for treatment. J Orofac Pain. 2001;15:93–105; discussion 106.
22. Turner JA, Dworkin SF. Screening for psychosocial risk factors in patients with chronic orofacial pain: recent advances. J Am Dent Assoc. 2004;135(8):1119–25.
23. NICE. Temporomandibular disorders (TMDs), clinical knowledge summary. 2016. Available from: https://cks.nice.org.uk/temporomandibular-disorders-tmds. Accessed 10 Spet 2018.
24. Cole F, Davies E, Jenner E. Live well with pain. 2018. Available from: https://my.livewellwithpain.co.uk/. Accessed 1 Nov 2018.
25. SungKun C, Kin GS, Lee JH. Psychometric evaluation of sleep hygiene index: a sample of patients with chronic pain. Health Qual Life Outcomes. 2013;11:213–9.
26. Moore C, Tang N. Getting a good night's sleep. Pain concern, Edinburgh. 2016. Available from: http://painconcern.org.uk/sleep/. Accessed 1 Nov 2018.
27. Sanders AE, Slade GD, Maixner W, Nackley AG, Diatchenko L, By K, Miller VE. Excess risk of temporomandibular disorder associated with cigarette smoking in young adults. J Pain. 2012;13(1):21–31.
28. Partland JM, Mitchell JA. Caffine and chronic back pain. Arch Phys Med Rehabil. 1997;78:61–3.

29. Wikoff D, et al. Systematic review of the potential adverse effects of caffeine consumption in healthy adults, pregnant women, adolescents, and children. Food Chem Toxicol. 2017;109:585–648.
30. Greene CS, Menchel HF. The use of oral appliances in the management of temporomandibular disorders. Oral Maxillofac Surg C N Am. 2018;30:265–77.
31. Turner JA, Mancl L, Aaron LA. Short- and long-term efficacy of brief cognitive-behavioural therapy for patients with chronic temporomandibular disorder pain: a randomized, controlled trial. Pain. 2006;121(3):181–94.
32. Aggarwal VR, Tickle M, Javidi H, et al. Reviewing the evidence: can cognitive behavioural therapy improve outcomes for patients with chronic orofacial pain? J Orofac Pain. 2010;24:163–71.
33. Aggarwal VR, Lovell K, Peters S, Javidi H, Joughin A, Goldthorpe J. Psychosocial interventions for the management of chronic orofacial pain. Cochrane Database Syst Rev. 2011;11:CD008456.
34. Mor N, Tang C, Blitzer A. Temporomandibular myofascial pain treated with Botulinum toxin injection. Toxins (Basel). 2015;7(8):2791–800.
35. Freund B, Schwartz M, Symington JM. Botulinum toxin: new treatment for temporomandibular disorders. Br J Oral Maxillofac Surg. 2000;38:466–71.
36. Silberstein SD, Gobel H, Jensen R, Elkind AH, Degryse R, Walcott JM, Turkel C. Botulinum toxin type A in the prophylactic treatment of chronic tension-type headache: a multicentre, double-blind, randomized, placebo-controlled, parallel-group study. Cephalalgia. 2006;26:790–800.
37. Ernberg M, Hedenberg-Magnusson B, List T, Svensson P. Efficacy of botulinum toxin type A for treatment of persistent myofascial TMD pain: a randomized, controlled, double-blind multicentre study. Pain. 2011;152(9):1988–96.
38. Kün-Darbois JD, Libouban H, Chappard D. Botulinum toxin in masticatory muscles of the adult rat induces bone loss at the condyle and alveolar regions of the mandible associated with a bone proliferation at a muscle enthesis. Bone. 2015;77:75–82.
39. NICE. Total prosthetic replacement of the Temporomandibular Joint. Interventional Procedure guidance 239. 2009. Available from: http://guidance.nice.org.uk/IPG329. Accessed 1 Oct 2018.

An Update on Headaches for the Dental Team

11

P. Chana and Tara Renton

Learning Objective

- The reader may wonder as to why there is a chapter on headaches for the dental team.
- Chronic primary headaches are common and often mimic dental and temporomandibular pain conditions.
- Chronic neurovascular pain, caused by primary headaches, is a main cause of orofacial pain particularly myalgia and arthralgia related to the temporomandibular joints.
- The reader will learn about differential diagnosis of chronic orofacial pain caused by primary headaches and how to differentiate them.
- The reader will also be alerted to sinister signs and when to advise their patient to seek further care.

Clinical Relevance
We aim to improve the knowledge of the dental team, in relation to primary headaches such that neurovascular pain can be differentiated from odontogenic causes of pain. We also aim to provide dental practitioners with the knowledge of how to initially manage the pain if it is neurovascular in origin in primary care.

P. Chana (✉) · T. Renton
King's College Hospital, London, UK
e-mail: pavneet.chana@nhs.net; tara.renton@kcl.ac.uk

11.1 Introduction

Pain in the head and neck region is often the driving factor for patients to seek care from the dental team. It is not rare for chronic orofacial pain conditions to manifest with similar symptoms to dental pain. This can often lead to a misdiagnosis and inappropriate treatment resulting in complications for both the clinician and the patient [1]. Diagnosis and management of these patients can be particularly challenging; however, a correct diagnosis is mandatory to ensure patient safety and care.

Headaches are predicted to affect up to 46% of the worldwide population, and they have been ranked as being one of the top 10 most disabling disorders [2]. Therefore, the implications to health care and patients should not be underestimated. The International Headache Society updated their classification in 2018 [3]. It is those that fall into the group of 'primary headaches' which are most relevant and may be encountered by the dental team; however, an awareness of the other types may also be beneficial. A general overview of the classification is shown in Table 11.1.

Due to the high number of patients who experience headaches and that the pain experienced may mimic dental pain, it is important that dental teams are able to correctly identify these disorders as they will be nonresponsive to routine care and if appropriate, may need referral on for urgent care. In general, dentists have a poor knowledge of headaches and often struggle with this. Two recent papers highlight the high proportion of patients who attended orofacial pain clinics who were suffering from primary headaches that ideally could have been signposted to neurologists sooner rather than experiencing years of pain and multiple inappropriate dental and ENT procedures [4, 5].

Table 11.1 An overview of the International Classification Disorders, third edition [3]

Primary headaches	1. Migraine
	2. Tension-type headache
	3. Trigeminal autonomic cephalalgias
	4. Other primary headache disorders
Secondary Headaches	5. Headache attributed to trauma or injury to head and/or neck
	6. Headache attributed to cranial and/or cervical vascular disorder
	7. Headache attributed to non-vascular intracranial disorder
	8. Headache attributed to a substance or its withdrawal
	9. Headache attributed to infection
	10. Headache attributed to disorder of homeostasis
	11. Headache or facial pain attributed to disorder of the cranium, neck, eyes, ears, nose, sinus
	12. Headache attributed to psychiatric disorder
Painful Cranial Neuropathies, Other Facial Pain and Other Headaches	13. Painful lesions of the cranial nerves and other facial pain
	14. Other headache disorders

11.2 Migraines

Migraines have been ranked as the third most prevalent disease in the world, so it is likely that dentists will encounter these patients [3]. Two main types exist, those with an aura and those without. Other types of migraines have been discussed in a previous paper suitable for dentists [2]. The diagnostic criteria for migraines have been defined by the International Headache Classification (Table 11.2). Migraines are more common in females, occur in all ages from childhood and have a unilateral distribution of pain (Fig. 11.1). They can last up to days and may be triggered by certain foods, alcohol, stress, the contraceptive pill or hormonal changes during the menstrual cycle [6]. Approximately, 20% of patients will experience an aura prior to the headache. Auras may be visual and examples include zigzag patterns, flashes of light or loss of vision. They may also be sensory such as tingling or numbness which can spread over the face, lips and tongue [7].

It is also of note to the reader that migraines may cause an increased risk of cardiovascular events, most commonly stroke, especially in women who smoke and take oestrogen supplements. They have also been linked to cerebrovascular disorders such as seizures. All of which should also be taken into account when managing these patients [8].

Table 11.2 Diagnostic criteria as defined by the International Headache Society [3]

Migraine without aura	A. At least five attacks fulfilling criteria B-D
	B. Headache attacks lasting 4–72 h
	C. Headache has at least two of the following four characteristics:
	1. Unilateral location
	2. Pulsating quality
	3. Moderate or severe pain intensity
	4. Aggravation by or causing avoidance of routine physical activity (e.g. walking or climbing stairs)
	D. During headache at least one of the following:
	1. Nausea and/or vomiting
	2. Photophobia or phonophobia
Migraine with aura	A. At least two attacks fulfilling criteria B and C
	B. One or more of the following fully reversible aura symptoms:
	1. Visual
	2. Sensory
	3. Speech and/or language
	4. Motor
	5. Brainstem
	6. Retinal
	C. At least three of the following characteristics:
	1. At least our aura symptom spreads gradually over >5 min
	2. Two or more aura symptoms occur in succession
	3. Each individual aura symptom lasts 5–60 min
	4. At least one aura symptom is unilateral
	5. At least one aura symptom is positive
	6. The aura is accompanied or followed within 60 min, by a headache

(continued)

Table 11.2 (continued)

Episodic tension-type headache	A. At least 10 episodes of headache occurring on <1 day/month on average (<12 days/year) and fulfilling the following criteria B. Lasting from 30 min to 7 days C. At least two of the following four characteristics: 　1. Bilateral location 　2. Pressing or tightening (non-pulsating) quality 　3. Mild or moderate intensity 　4. Not aggravated by routine physical activity such as walking or climbing stairs D. Both of the following: 　1. No nausea or vomiting 　2. No more than one of photophobia or phonophobia
Chronic tension-type headache	A. Headache occurring on >15 days/month on average for >3 months (>180 days/year, fulfilling criteria B-D. B. Lasting hours to days, or unremitting. C-D. As above
Cluster headaches	A. At least five attacks fulfilling criteria B-D B. Severe or very severe unilateral orbital, supraorbital and/or temporal pain lasted 15–180 min– when untreated C. Either or both of the following: 　1. At least one of the following symptoms or signs ipsilateral to the headache: 　　(a) Conjunctival injection and/or lacrimation 　　(b) Nasal congestion and/or rhinorrhoea 　　(c) Eyelid oedema 　　d) Forehead and facial sweating 　　e) Miosis and/or ptosis 　2. A sense of restlessness or agitation D. Occurring with a frequency between one every other day and eight per day

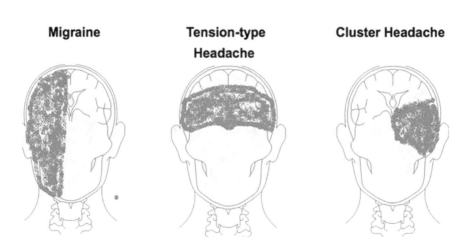

Migraine　　**Tension-type Headache**　　**Cluster Headache**

Fig. 11.1 Pattern of distribution of pain in primary headaches [2]

The patient should also be questioned sensitively about depression and anxiety; both of these have been linked to migraines, likely due to the common pain receptors involved in both. A presence of these disorders has been shown to reduce compliance with prescribed medications and advice on management [8].

11.2.1 Common Differential Diagnoses

- Odontogenic Pain.
- Sinus Pain.
- Temporomandibular joint disorder.

Migraines most commonly cause pain in the V1 distribution, but they may also cause pain in the V2 and V3 distribution, occasionally independent of pain in V1 [1, 9]. Due to the distribution of pain presenting in the V2 and V3 region, dentists may be confused and misdiagnose the pain has having a dental or sinus origin. Migraines presenting with isolated facial pain in V2 and/or V3 region is considered extremely rare and its phenotype has not been described in full.

There is also a well-established link between temporomandibular joint disorders and migraines due to the similar neurophysiological processes involved in both conditions [10]. Although this may complicate the diagnosis of the patients' pain, if this is found to be the case it is suggested that they should be managed using a simultaneous approach to both conditions, rather than managing each OFP condition separately [11].

11.2.2 Treatment

11.2.2.1 General Dental Practitioners

General dental practitioners may give patients advice on acute treatment which aims to offer patients a reduction in the pain and other symptoms experienced with a treatment goal of reducing the disability associated with migraines. The evidence favours NSAIDS (aspirin, diclofenac, ibuprofen, naproxen), triptans, ergotamine derivatives and opioids such as butorphanol. A combination of medications is also well supported in the literature with a triptan and NSADS being more effective than pairing a triptan with paracetamol [12]. Despite the evidence supporting the benefits of using opioids in migraines, NICE doesn't recommend that they should be prescribed to patients due to side effects and risk of dependence [12]. Of note, NSAIDs can result in gastrointestinal and cardiovascular adverse effects so they should be used with caution. In addition, triptans should be avoided in patients with coronary artery disease, poorly controlled hypertension and other peripheral vascular diseases. Newer medications are being developed to overcome the vascular contraindications of triptans.

11.2.2.2   Specialist Referral Treatment

Treatment to prevent migraines, normally provided by a specialist in the field, is considered based on the frequency of migraines experienced and the level of disability. The following medications have an established evidence base for their efficacy in preventing migraines: antiepileptic drugs, triptans and hypotensives including; beta-blockers (metoprolol, propranolol, timolol). In comparison, antidepressants and other beta-blockers such as atenolol may also be considered, but there is less evidence to support the use of these drugs [13]. Although gabapentin may have been previously recommended, guidelines updated in 2019 by NICE have advised that it should not be offered to patients [1, 12].

Emerging treatments for the prevention of migraines include injectable therapies which can be administered both subcutaneously and intravenously such as botulinum toxin A and monoclonal antibodies, but there are still questions over their long-term safety [13]. Neuromodulation is also an emerging active treatment for migraines which may be suitable for patients who are not responding to drug therapy or have contraindications [13, 14].

Biobehavioural therapy such as cognitive behaviour therapy should also not be ignored. In more recent years, there is a growing body of evidence to support their use in chronic pain as well as migraines [13]. Further evidence has shown that using these techniques alongside drug therapy has been shown to be more effective than using drugs alone [15].

11.3   Tension-Type Headaches

Tension-type headaches (TTH) are the most common type of headache experienced by patients and thought to affect up to 78% of the population [2, 3]. Their diagnostic criteria can also be seen in Table 11.2. The mild to moderate pain tends to be bilateral and a pressing or tightening pain (Fig. 11.1). This is a non-pulsating pain, in comparison to a migraine which often has a pulsating type pain [2]. TTH can be further classified into episodic and chronic which has been elaborated on in Table 11.2. In very rare cases, a tension headache can show similar symptoms to concerning conditions such as a subarachnoid haemorrhage, TIA or stroke.

11.3.1   Common Differential Diagnoses

• Temporomandibular joint disorders including headache attributed to TMD.

The pain experienced during a TTH is commonly confused and therefore diagnosed as temporomandibular joint disorder pain caused by bruxism as often in both conditions the temporalis may be tender to palpate [16].

The relationship between bruxism and TTH should be acknowledged by the dental team and recent evidence supports an association between the two [17]. A proposed modern theory is that TTH may result from referred pain from trigger points in head and shoulder muscles. Bruxism may be a factor in the development of trigger points in the head and neck region. It is these trigger points are responsible for central sensitisation which has noted to be present in TTH [17]. Further to this, patients who suffer from TTH also report heavier tooth contact, muscle tension, stress and more pain in their head region [18].

11.3.2 Treatment

11.3.2.1 General Dental Practitioners
The mild to moderate pain experienced by patients can be managed with analgesics which may be prescribed by their general dental practitioner if deemed suitable. The effectiveness of analgesics is reduced if the patient frequently experiences TTH. As a first-line treatment, acetaminophen (paracetamol) may be prescribed which is favourable due to the reduced gastric side effects and as a second-line ibuprofen can be prescribed.

11.3.2.2 Specialist Referral Treatment
For patients suffering from chronic TTH, drug therapy can be used to reduce the frequency and severity of headaches. Tricyclic antidepressants are most widely used, with amitriptyline found to be the most effective [19, 20]. Mirtazapine may also be used. Other types of antidepressants such as SSRI and tetracyclic are not indicated in these patients. Botulinum toxin A has also been licenced for use; however, there is a lot of conflicting evidence supporting this as a treatment modality and further research is needed to be undertaken in this area [20].

As with migraines, a combination of pharmacological and non-pharmacological treatments (physical and/or psychological therapy such as CBT) has been shown to be more effective than using one treatment alone [19, 20]. Although the links to bruxism have been discussed, dentists should not routinely use an occlusal splint to treat TTH due to the lack of supporting evidence as a treatment modality [19, 21].

11.4   Trigeminal Autonomic Cephalalgias

The trigeminal autonomic cephalalgias (TACs) are composed of a group of short-lasting and unilateral headaches that also present with cranial autonomic features which are lateralised and ipsilateral to the headache [22]. These include cluster headaches, paroxysmal hermicrania, short-lasting unilateral neuralgia headache attacks and hemicrania continua [3]. Despite these headaches being rare, these patients may present in a dental setting and due to the extremely debilitating nature of these headaches it is important that they can be appropriately managed.

The presenting pain is an intense unilateral pain with neuralgic multiple stabbing events which lasts several hours and spontaneously regresses leaving the patient with pain-free interludes. The pain episodes often occur several times a day at the same times usually early mornings and clusters of pain most commonly occurring in spring and autumn [1]. There are associated autonomic signs which include: drooping of the eyelid (ptosis), redness of the cheek or eye, pupil constriction (meiosis) and nasal congestion. The presence of nasal congestion often leads patients to seek ENT opinions resulting in inappropriate ENT procedures.

The rest of this article will focus on updating the reader on cluster headaches as this is the most common form of TACs, the other forms of TACs are covered in previous papers aimed at dentists [2, 22].

11.5   Cluster Headaches

These are usually unilateral and located to around or above the eye (Fig. 11.1). The pain is severe and has a number of presentations such as burning, tightening or throbbing. The diagnostic criteria can also be seen in Table 11.2. They may also be further classified into being episodic or chronic in nature. If the patient experiences multiple episodes of cluster headaches with breaks of less than 3 months, then they are classified as chronic. Triggering factors include alcohol, nitrate containing food, nitro-glycerine and strong odours such as pain or nail vanish [22].

The pain experienced by patients is often described as the worst pain they have ever experienced, and cluster headaches have been termed 'suicidal headaches' as patients have been known to develop suicidal thoughts [2]. Cluster headaches more commonly affect men and those who are over the age of 50 [6].

Interestingly, these patients most commonly seek help initially from dentists, and there are multiple studies which have found inappropriate treatment on patients in an attempt to relieve the pain of misdiagnosed TACs [1, 22].

11.5.1 Common Differential Diagnoses

- Odontogenic pain.
- Temporomandibular joint disorder.
- Trigeminal neuralgia.

Due to the episodic pattern of pain and areas commonly affected by TACs, they are often misdiagnosed as toothaches. During the attacks by themselves, pain has been known to be experienced in the teeth and jaw [22, 23]. The jaw pain experienced may be confused with temporomandibular joint disorder.

11.5.2 Treatment

Although the management of cluster headaches is out of the remit of general dental practitioners, it is useful that dentists are aware of the management. As with other types of headaches, the management of these patients is subdivided into prevention and acute management.

For acute management, the evidence supports subcutaneous or intranasal sumatriptan, intranasal zolmitriptan and oxygen [24]. For prevention, verapamil is most commonly used. Lithium, melatonin and topiramate may also be used, but the evidence is more limited regarding their use [24, 25]. Whilst waiting for preventative treatment to work, prednisolone may be prescribed. Due to the side effects of steroids, a unilateral greater occipital nerve block may be performed using either lidocaine or methylprednisolone which has effects lasting up to 4 weeks [2, 24].

11.6 Sinister Headaches

Recent onset of a headache or sudden worsening of headache in a middle-aged patient is rare. If it is associated with sensory or motor neuropathy, nausea, loss of consciousness or other aberrant signs immediate referral to the patients' general medical practitioner or advice to attend A&E is advised, as exclusion of ischaemic or haemorrhagic stroke and or neoplasia must be undertaken urgently. Exclusion of a recent history of head injury must be excluded and any patient with comorbid poorly controlled or undiagnosed hypertension may indicate a potential stroke risk.

11.6.1 Misdiagnosis

Common features of neurovascular pain which may mimic odontogenic and complicate diagnosis include [26]:

- A deep, throbbing, spontaneous pain which may last up to a few days and be pulsatile in nature may be experienced, similar to how pulpal pain is described.
- The pain is predominantly unilateral.
- Headache is often accompanied by a toothache.
- Periodic and recurrent nature of pain.
- Some autonomic signs may bear a resemblance to a dental abscess such as oedema of the eyelids.

11.7 Differentiating Between Neurovascular and Odontogenic Pain

There are a number of ways in which the conditions described in this paper can be differentiated from odontogenic pain. Table 11.3 gives an overview of the differentiating features between neurovascular and odontogenic pain to aid general dental practitioners in correct diagnosis [27].

Table 11.3 Differentiating between neurovascular and odontogenic pain [27]

	Migraine	Tension-type headaches	Cluster headaches	Acute pulpal pain	Chronic pulpal pain	Periodontal pain
Pain Type	Pulsating	Pressing, Tightening, Non-pulsating	Orbital	Throbbing, Aching	Tender, Aching	Tender, Aching
Pain severity	Moderate to severe	Mild to moderate	Severe	Mild to severe	Mild	Mild
Location	Frontotemporal Unilateral	Frontal Bilateral	Orbital Unilateral	Tooth Unilateral	Tooth Unilateral	Tooth, Gingivae Unilateral
Duration	4–72 h	30 min–7 days	15–180 min	Seconds to daily	Constant	Varies
Frequency	1/month	1–30/month	1–8/day	Variable	Daily	Daily
Autonomic Features	Yes	No	Yes	No	No	No
Triggers	Stress, food, alcohol, hormones, lack of sleep	Stress, muscle tension	Alcohol, nitrates	Electrical or thermal stimulation, percussion of tooth	Varies	Lateral pressure, apical pressure

A good knowledge base of the signs and symptoms of primary headaches, as well as those related to odontogenic pain will allow an initial diagnosis from the pain history provided from the patient. Specifically, the way the patient describes the type of pain, the location of pain, the triggers of pain, the duration and frequency of the pain will all help form an initial diagnosis just from the patient's history (Table 11.3). It is also imperative that the general dental practitioner establishes whether any autonomic features have also been experienced. This will be a key distinguishing factor supporting a neurovascular cause of pain. Secondary to this, a clinical examination supported with radiographs will allow dental pathology to be identified which will help dentists form a definitive diagnosis.

11.8 Conclusion

Headaches may present in various ways, and it is likely that these patients will present to dentists, especially as the pain may be experienced in their teeth and jaws. Dentists have a responsibility to correctly diagnose pain in the head and neck region. If headaches are suspected an appropriate referral to an OFP service or neurology clinic is favoured as opposed to unnecessary irreversible dental treatment.

Acknowledgement Reproduced with kind permission of the publishers of Dental Update, Mark Allen Dentistry Media Ltd.

References

1. Renton T. Tooth-related pain or not? Headache. 2020;60(1):235–46.
2. Chong MS, Renton T. Pain part 10: headaches. Dent Update. 2016;43:448–60.
3. The International Headache society. The international classification of headache disorders, 3rd edition. Cephalagia. 2018;38(1):1–211.
4. Lambru G, Elias LA, Yakkaphan P, Renton T. Migraine presenting as isolated facial pain: a prospective clinical analysis of 58 cases. Cephalalgia. 2020;40(11):1250–4.
5. Wei DY, Moreno-Ajona D, Renton T, Goadsby PJ. Trigeminal autonomic cephalalgias presenting in a multidisciplinary tertiary orofacial pain clinic. J Headahe Pain. 2019;20:69.
6. Coulthard P, Horner K, Sloan P, Theaker E. Oral and maxillofacial surgery, radiology, pathology and oral medicine. 3rd ed. London: Churchill Livingstone; 2013.
7. Weatherall MW. The diagnosis and treatment of chronic migraine. Ther Adv Chronic Dis. 2015;6(3):115–23.
8. Nixdord DR, Velly AM, Alonson AA. Neurovascular pains: implications of migraine for the oral and maxillofacial surgeon. Oral Maxillofac Surg Clin North Am. 2008;20(2):221–vii. https://doi.org/10.1016/j.coms.2007.12.008.
9. Yoon MS, Mueller D, Hansen N, Poitz F, Slomke M, Dommes P, Diener HC, Katsarava Z, Obermann M. Prevalence of facial pain in population-based study. Cephalagia. 2009;30(1):92–6.
10. Smith JG, Karamat A, Melek L, Jayakumar S, Renton T. The differential impact of neuromuscular musculoskeletal and neurovascular orofacial pain on psychosocial function. J Oral Pathol Med. 2020;49(6):538–46.
11. Speciali JG, Dach F. Temporomandibular dysfunction and headache disorder. Headache. 2015;55(S1):72–83. https://doi.org/10.1111/head.12515.
12. NICE. Migraine. National Institute for Health and Care Excellence. 2019. https://cks.nice.org.uk/migraine#!references.
13. American Headache Society. The American Headache Society Position Statement on Integrating New Migraine Treatments into Clinical Practice. Headache. 2019;59(1):1–18. https://doi.org/10.1111/head.13456.
14. Puledda F, Messina R, Goadsby PJ. An update on migraine: current understanding and future directions. J Neurol. 2017;264(9):2031–9. https://doi.org/10.1007/s00415-017-8434-y.
15. Harris P, Loveman E, Clegg A, Easton S, Berry N. Systematic review of cognitive behavioural therapy for the management of headaches and migraines in adults. Br J Pain. 2015;9:213–24.
16. May A. Hints on diagnosing and treating headache. Dtsch Arztebl Int. 2018;115(17):299–308. https://doi.org/10.3238/arztebl.2018.0299.
17. De Luca Canto G, Singh V, Bigal ME, Major PW, Flores-Mir C. Association between tension-type headache and migraine with sleep bruxism: a systematic review. Headache. 2014;54(9):1460–9. https://doi.org/10.1111/head.12446.
18. Glaros AG, Urban D, Locke J. Headache and temporomandibular disorders: Evidence for diagnostic and behavioural overlap. Cephalalgia. 2007;27:542–9.
19. Jensen RH. Tension-type headache – The normal and most prevalent headache. Headache. 2018;58(2):339–45. https://doi.org/10.1111/head.13067.
20. Yu S, Han X. Update of chronic tension-type headache. Curr Pain Headache Rep. 2015;19:469. https://doi.org/10.1007/s11916-014-0469-5.
21. List T, Jensen R. TMD: old ideas and new concepts. Cephalalgia. 2017;37(7):692–704. https://doi.org/10.1177/0333102416686302.
22. Baker NA, Matharu M, Renton T. Pain part 9: trigeminal autonomic cephalalgias. Dent Update. 2016;43(4):340–52.
23. Bahra A, May A, Goadsby PJ. Cluster headache: a prospective clinical study with diagnostic implications. Neurology. 2002;58(3):354–61.

24. Wei DY, Khalil M, Goadsby P. Managing cluster headache. Pract Neurol. 2019;19:521–8.
25. Kingston WS, Dodlick DW. Treatment of cluster headache. Ann Indian Acad Neurol. 2018;21(Suppl 1):S9–S15. https://doi.org/10.4103/aian.AIAN_17_18.
26. Garg N, Garg A. Textbook of endodontics. 3rd ed. London: JP Medical Ltd.; 2003.
27. Balasubramaniam R, Turner LN, Fischer D, Klasser GD, Okeson JP. Non-odontogenic toothache revisited. Open J Stomatol. 2011;1:92–102.

Rhinosinusitis Update

12

Claire Hopkins

Learning Objectives

- The reader may wonder as to why there is a chapter on rhinosinusitis for the dental team.
- Rhinosinusitis is common and often mimics dental and orofacial pain.
- Chronic pain in the sinuses, is more commonly caused by migraine than chronic rhinosinusitis.
- Caused by migraine in up to 90% of cases.
- The reader will learn about differential diagnosis of rhinosinusitis and how dental disease may impact on sinus health.
- The reader will also be alerted to sinister signs and when to advise their patient to seek further care.

Rhinosinusitis is a common condition, affecting more than one in ten adults. This article will review current management strategies. While multi-factorial in aetiology, odontogenic rhinosinusitis is an important subgroup that is often misdiagnosed and recalcitrant to management. Patients with rhinosinusitis often report facial pain, but when it is severe, and mismatched in severity to other sinonasal symptoms, facial migraine should be suspected. Finally, the risks of implantation in the setting of maxillary sinus mucosal thickening and the need for ENT referral in such cases will be discussed.

C. Hopkins (✉)
King's College London and ENT Department, Guy's and St Thomas' Hospitals, London, UK

12.1   Introduction

Rhinosinusitis is a condition of inflammation of the nose and paranasal sinuses. Rhinosinusitis is divided into acute and chronic forms. In acute rhinosinusitis (ARS) symptoms resolve within 12 weeks (although usually within 4 weeks) and often have an infective aetiology, while in chronic rhinosinusitis (CRS), symptoms last more than 12 weeks without complete resolution with multiple potential aetiologies, which may include inflammation, infection and obstruction of sinus ventilation [1]. CRS is subcategorised into chronic rhinosinusitis with nasal polyps (CRSwNP) and without nasal polyps (CRSsNP), based on visualisation of polyps on rhinoscopy or endoscopy. In a worldwide population study, 10.9% of UK adults reported CRS symptoms [2].

12.2   Acute Rhinosinusitis

Acute rhinosinusitis is usually caused by a viral infection and is usually self-limiting. NICE guidance [3] advocates avoidance of antibiotic prescribing unless symptoms persists for more than 10 days, or if the patient has a high risk of complications or is systemically very unwell. First choice antibiotics in such cases would be co-amoxiclav or doxycycline. A large number of high quality randomised trials support restricting usage of antibiotics [4]—although antibiotics can shorted resolution of the episode, only 1 in 20 benefits, while 1 in 8 will develop side effects of antibiotic treatment. Despite this evidence, ARS accounts for over 20% of antibiotic prescriptions, with antibiotics being issued in over 90% of consultations for ARS [5].

12.3   Chronic Rhinosinusitis

In contrast, most chronic rhinosinusitis (CRS) is associated with inflammation as the primary abnormality, with preservation of drainage pathways, although acute infective exacerbations may occur. It is thought that the persistent inflammation found in CRS is due to a dysfunctional host–environment, with abnormal responses of the mucosa to a wide variety of microbes and irritants. Targeting inflammation is therefore central to treatment options, rather than targeting the microbes or simple drainage procedures. This is reflected in the move away from antibiotic treatment in chronic disease. CRS has been shown to have significant impact on quality of life (QOL) with symptoms such as nasal obstruction, nasal discharge, facial pain, anosmia and sleep disturbance.

Diagnosis of CRS is made by the presence of two or more persistent symptoms for at least 12 weeks without complete resolution, one of which should be nasal congestion/obstruction/nasal discharge and/or facial pain/pressure /headache or loss/reduction in smell. Symptoms must be accompanied by endoscopic evidence of mucoprulent secretions, polyps or oedema or radiological evidence of disease, as a symptom-based diagnosis alone has high sensitivity but poor specificity—only 50% meeting the symptom-based definition have supporting objective signs of disease [6].

First-line treatment in CRS usually includes a trial of intranasal corticosteroids (INCS) and saline irrigation. INCS have been shown to be effective in a large number of randomised trials, with a low incidence of adverse effects [7]. This treatment is the same for both CRS with and without polyps although steroid drops may be considered for patients with polyps to help achieve better nasal entry. Patients should be advised that steroid sprays work best when used regularly and do not perform well imply as a rescue medication. It is important that compliance is encouraged. Daily large volume saline irrigation should be recommended [8], and a number of positive pressure squeeze bottles or irrigations jugs are available commercially.

Antibiotics are not recommended for routine management of CRS, except in the setting of an acute exacerbation. Patients with CRS often receive multiple courses of oral antibiotics that may increase risk of antibiotic resistance. There is little evidence for any benefit of short-term oral antibiotics in CRS. There is weak evidence for the use of a 12-week course of a low-dose macrolide [9], in highly selected patients with CRSsNP, although there is a small risk of cardiac toxicity [10].

Patients who fail to achieve sufficient symptomatic control with medical treatment may be considered for surgery. Surgical intervention typically involves endoscopic sinus surgery to open and ventilate sinuses, restore normal mucociliary functioning and improve access to topical steroids (see Fig. 12.1). 'Functional' endoscopic surgery focuses on opening the ostiomeatal complex, and the key drainage pathway of the maxillary, anterior ethmoid and frontal sinuses in the middle meatus. Inferior meatal antrostomies and sinus wash-outs are no longer performed as they do not improve mucociliary drainage. In more extensive sinus disease, or in the presence of tumours, extended procedures may be undertaken, including complete ethmoidectomy, sphenoidotomy, medial maxillectomy and median drainage of the frontal sinuses. Use of navigation systems may facilitate surgical dissection in the setting of complex anatomical variations or revision cases. Nasal polyp removal, surgery to manage underlying nasal abnormalities such as septal deviation or turbinate hypertrophy may also be performed. Studies have shown greater benefits in surgery performed at an early stage in the disease process [11]. Currently, commissioning restrictions and delays in primary care result in 50% patients who currently undergo endoscopic sinus surgery waiting for more than 5 years from the onset of symptoms of CRS, potentially missing the window of greatest benefit. Although up to 15% of patients with CRSwNP require revision surgery over a 5-year period, surgery improves the effectiveness of ongoing topical therapy and achieves significant improvements in disease-related quality of life that is maintained long term [12].

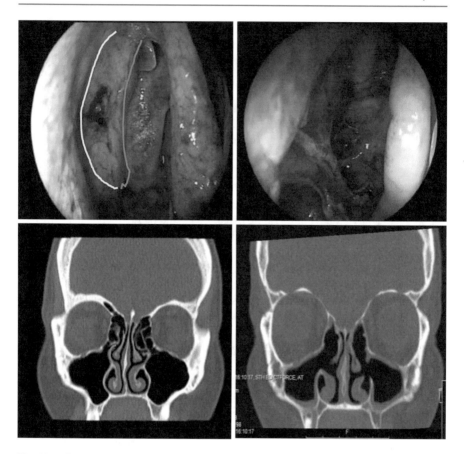

Fig. 12.1 Preoperative CT and endoscopy images shown on the left. The cleft between the free posterior margin of the uncinate process, marked in blue on the CT and outlined in blue on the endoscopy image below, and the ethmoid bulla (*) is known as the hiatus semilunaris, and key to the drainage of the anterior ethmoid, maxillary and frontal sinuses. This common drainage pathway is called the ostiomeatal complex. During functional endoscopic sinus surgery, the uncinate is removed along its anterior margin (marked in yellow) to expose the maxillary sinus ostium and the ethmoidal bulla and partitions are removed to remove any obstruction to sinus drainage and allow topical access to the sinuses. On the right, the postoperative CT shows the widely opened sinus cavities; on the endoscopic image, the frontal recess (F) skull base and maxillary sinuses are exposed

12.4   Facial Pain and Rhinosinusitis

Facial pain is reported by 50% patients with CRS, but is infrequently severe and usually mirrors the severity of other nasal symptoms. When pain is severe, and the main presenting symptom, then a careful history for migraines should be taken, and key features of the pain should be elicited. Indeed, facial pain, particularly if reported as 'throbbing 'or associated with light sensitivity, has a significant negative predictive value in diagnosing CRS; its presence makes CRS LESS likely [13]. This is also found when there is a mismatch in the severity of facial pain and aural fullness compared with the overall severity of nasal symptoms [14], or a mismatch in the severity of symptoms and endoscopy and radiological scores [15].

Facial migraine is commonly misdiagnosed by both patients and physicians as chronic or recurrent acute rhinosinusitis; it typically presents with severe pain over the paranasal sinuses and is often associated with tenderness over the glabellar area and may be accompanied by congestion and clear rhinorrhoea. Pain is usually intermittent, but episodes can be frequently and are often exacerbated by overuse of codeine analgesia. Often patients are given repeated courses of antibiotics, but with limited effectiveness. Of patients who met IHS criteria for migraines, 84% of patients reported sinus pressure, 82% reported pain in the sinus areas, 63% reported nasal congestion and 40% reported rhinorrhoea at the time of their initial consultation [16]—it is therefore easy to understand why the symptoms are thought to arise in the sinuses. Vasodilation, occurring as a downstream effect of migraines may cause sinonasal symptoms, may be relieved by use of decongestants, thereby falsely re-affirming the diagnosis of sinogenic headache [17]. In a large series of nearly 3000 patients with self-diagnosed sinus headache, 88% were found to have migraine and 8% tension headaches [18]; most had bifrontal and bimaxillary pain [18]. In another study, 58% of patients with self-diagnosed sinus headache who had negative CT and endoscopy were found to have migraine [19].

Mehle et al. observed, in a cohort of 35 patients affected by self-referred 'sinus headache' that 74.3% satisfied International Headache Society (IHS) criteria for migraine [20]; interestingly, the sinus radiological score (measured using a Lund-Mackay scale) did not differentiate between migrainous and non-migrainous headaches, with mild mucosal thickening and anatomical variants being also found in migraineurs. This highlights one of the diagnostic challenges; a limitation of CT imaging is that abnormalities are found in up to 39% asymptomatic patients, and the mean Lund-Mackay score in a normal population is 4 [21]. CT changes alone therefore have limited specificity and should be viewed in association with presenting symptoms (see Table 12.1 for the HIS criteria for rhinogenic headaches).

Recurrent acute rhinosinusitis is actually very rare, and facial migraine should certainly be considered in the setting of frequent intermittent episodes of facial pain in the absence of mucopurulent discharge. Often, endoscopy or a CT scan performed during an acute episode is required to differentiate between the two, as imaging performed in between episodes. In one study of patients referred to tertiary care thought to be having recurrent episodes of ARS, CT performed at baseline was normal at baseline and remained so when repeated the time of an acute episode, excluding recurrent ARS in 96% [22]. 47% were ultimately diagnosed with rhinitis, 37% with migraine and 12.5% with otherwise unspecified facial pain. Correct and early diagnosis of migrainous headache is important, both to achieve adequate symptom control and to avoid unnecessary and often repeated courses of medical, and sometimes surgical, treatment. One patient referred to my practice with 'recalcitrant recurrent acute sinusitis' had undergone seven sinus procedures despite no evidence of mucosal thickening or other radiological signs of CRS, but made an excellent response to treatment for facial migraine.

Table 12.1 Diagnostic criteria for headache attributed to rhinosinusitis. Headache Classification Committee of the International Headache Society (IHS), the International Classification of Headache Disorders. third edition. *Cephalalgia* 2018;38:1–211

Attributed to acute rhinosinusitis	Attributed to chronic or recurring rhinosinusitis
A. Any headache fulfilling criterion C	A. Any headache fulfilling criterion C
B. Clinical, nasal endoscopic and/or imaging evidence of acute rhinosinusitis	B. Clinical, nasal endoscopic and/or imaging evidence of current or past infection or other inflammatory process within the paranasal sinuses

C. Evidence of causation demonstrated by at least 2 of the following:
1. Headache is developed in temporal relation to the onset of rhinosinusitis
2. Either or both of the following:
  (a) Headache as significantly worsened in parallel with worsening of the rhinosinusitis
  (b) Headache as significantly improved or resolved in parallel with improvement in or resolution of the rhinosinusitis
3. Headache is exacerbated by pressure applied over the paranasal sinuses
4. In the case of unilateral rhinosinusitis, headache is localised and ipsilateral to it
	C. Evidence of causation demonstrated by at least 2 of the following:
	1. Headache as developed in temporal relation to the onset of chronic rhinosinusitis;
	2. Headache waxes and wanes in parallel with the degree of sinus congestion and other symptoms of the chronic rhinosinusitis;
	3. Headache is exacerbated by pressure applied over the paranasal sinuses;
	4. In the case of unilateral rhinosinusitis, headache is localised and ipsilateral to it.

D. Not better accounted for/by another ICHD-III diagnosis	D. Not better accounted for/by another ICHD-III diagnosis

Within specialist clinics, 'upfront' CT should be considered in patients with negative endoscopy before prescribing 'maximal medical therapy' and reinforcing a diagnosis of sinus disease [23]. Primary care and dental practitioners should similarly avoid reinforcing patient perceptions of a sinogenic headache unless there is clear supporting evidence on examination or radiology.

12.5   Odontogenic Sinusitis

Odontogenic sinusitis, where a dental origin is identified clinically, radiologically, or suggested by anaerobic predominance on culture, may present as an acute or chronic picture. It is estimated that 10% of all sinusitis cases have an odontogenic cause and up to 40% of recalcitrant maxillary sinusitis cases [24, 25]. The incidence of odontogenic sinusitis appears to be increasing [26], possibly related to the rising rates of dental implantation [27]. Only 50% of patients have a history of previous dental surgery or known periapical disease [28], and as dental pain is often absent, odontogenic disease may present directly to ENT, where the diagnosis can be easily missed [29]. Foul-smelling unilateral mucopurulent nasal discharge should raise suspicion of an odontogenic sinusitis. Facial pain and pressure, nasal obstruction and post-nasal drip may also be reported.

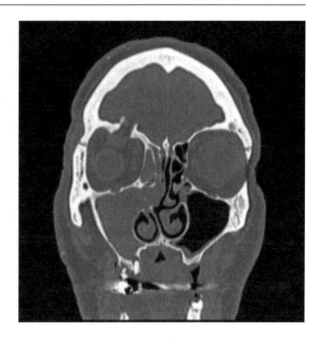

Fig. 12.2 Odontogenic sinusitis periapical lucency and extensive opacification of the ipsilateral sinuses. The patient developed orbital cellulitis and an extradural collection secondary to the odontogenic infection

Anterior rhinoscopy and endoscopy, which may reveal mucopurulence and oedema in the middle meatus, and dental examination, are helpful in making the diagnosis but radiological imaging is essential. CT is considered the gold standard (Fig. 12.2), as high rates of false negatives are reported with periapical radiography [30]. Ideally if CBCT is used, the field of view should include the ostiomeatal complex, the drainage pathway of the maxillary sinus found in the superomedial aspect of the sinus.

Anaerobic streptococci, Gram-negative bacilli and enterobacteriae are the most commonly isolated microbes [31] although infections are usually polymicrobial.

Initial medical management should include nasal decongestants and appropriate broad-spectrum antibiotics, such as co-amoxiclav or clindamycin. The dental origin should be addressed. While may patients will settle with conservative management, sinus surgery will likely be required in up to 50% of cases [32]; this is more likely if there is a history of preceding dental procedure (particularly implantation) or if there is obstruction to the drainage of the maxillary sinus.

12.6   Management of the Sinuses Prior to Dental Implantation

No doubt driven by wish to avoid iatrogenic odontogenic sinusitis, an increasing number of patients appear to being referred to the NHS to investigate incidental findings in the maxillary sinus found on CBCT prior to implantation.

Fig. 12.3 Right-sided maxillary mucous retention cyst

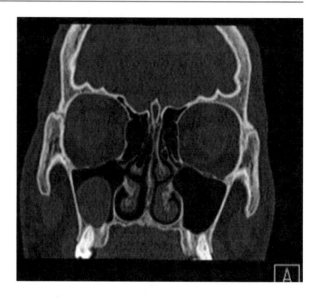

There are currently few published studies upon which to guide management in such cases although the British Rhinological Society are in the process of developing a consensus document.

One of the most common incidental findings is a mucosal retention cyst (Fig. 12.3); these are found in a third of CT scans performed for non-rhinological conditions are not a manifestation of rhinosinusitis [33]. They are rarely symptomatic and have a high recurrence rate after marsupialisation, and therefore treatment is not required.

Mucosal thickening is also common in the absence of sinus disease. A study of patients undergoing sinus imaging for non-sinusitis causes found that only 25% had no mucosal thickening, with a mean Lund-Mackay score (a staging system that quantifies the amount of mucosal thickening on a scale of 0–24) of 4.26 [34]. Dental literature defines rhinosinusitis based on radiological thickening of the mucosa of >2mm [35], but this definition has poor specificity and will include many healthy asymptomatic patients.

The presence of mucosal thickening on CT has been shown to not affect the success of dental implants. In one study, with strict inclusion criteria, 29 CBCT scans being evaluated prior to dental implantation. Of these, 6.9% had minimal thickening (1–2 mm), 20.7% of cases had moderate thickening (2–5 mm) and 65.5% had severe thickening (>5 mm). There was a 100% success rate of the implants with no loss of implantation or infection [36]. This is also supported by a study by Jungner et al. in 2014, whereby radiographic signs of sinus pathology, opacification, polyp-like structures, and thickening of the sinus membrane, were not correlated to implant survival [37]. A key feature is whether the drainage pathway of the maxillary sinus, the ostiomeatal complex is patent; this should be included in the field of view on cone beam imaging if rhinosinusitis is suspected. If the drainage pathway is unobstructed, there is only mild mucosal thickening and if the patient is asymptomatic, there is no need for ENT assessment. In all other cases, onward ENT referral should be made, with

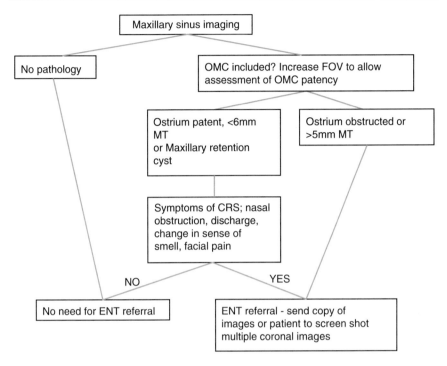

Fig. 12.4 Management algorithm for mucosal thickening discovered during pre-implantation planning

transfer of the appropriate imaging. As NHS systems are often are unable to open CDs or import images, it can be helpful to ask the patient to take pictures of relevant images on their smartphone. A treatment algorithm is proposed in Fig. 12.4.

12.7 Conclusions

Rhinosinusitis is a common chronic condition requiring early, correct diagnosis, medical management and at times surgical intervention. Radiological imaging may be required to distinguish between facial migraine in the setting of normal endoscopy.

Severe facial pain is an uncommon feature of chronic rhinosinusitis and should prompt consideration of neuropathic causes.

Odontogenic sinusitis should be considered with unilateral rhinosinusitis, and expedient management of the dental cause will result in resolution in over 50% of cases.

Mild mucosal thickening and mucous retention cysts in the maxillary sinus are not contraindications to dental implantation, but ENT assessment is advised if the sinus drainage is obstructed.

Acknowledgement Reproduced with kind permission of the publishers of Dental Update, Mark Allen Dentistry Media Ltd.

References

1. Fokkens WJ, Lund VJ, Mullol J, et al. European Position Paper on Rhinosinusitis and Nasal Polyps 2012. Rhinol Suppl. 2012:3; preceding table of contents, 1–298
2. Hastan D, Fokkens WJ, Bachert C, et al. Chronic rhinosinusitis in Europe—an underestimated disease. A GA(2)LEN study. Allergy. 2011;66:1216–23. https://doi.org/10.1111/j.1398-9995 .2011.02646.x.
3. Guidance N. Sinusitis (acute): antimicrobial prescribing. 2017.
4. Lemiengre MB, van Driel ML, Merenstein D, et al. Antibiotics for acute rhinosinusitis in adults. Cochrane Database Syst Rev. 2018;9:CD006089. https://doi.org/10.1002/14651858. CD006089.pub5.
5. Ashworth M, Charlton J, Ballard K, et al. Variations in antibiotic prescribing and consultation rates for acute respiratory infection in UK general practices 1995-2000. Br J Gen Pract. 2005;55:603–8.
6. Bhattacharyya N, Lee LN. Evaluating the diagnosis of chronic rhinosinusitis based on clinical guidelines and endoscopy. Otolaryngol Head Neck Surg. 2010;143:147–51. https://doi. org/10.1016/j.otohns.2010.04.012.
7. Chong LY, Head K, Hopkins C, et al. Intranasal steroids versus placebo or no intervention for chronic rhinosinusitis. Cochrane Database Syst Rev. 2016;4:CD011996. https://doi. org/10.1002/14651858.CD011996.pub2.
8. Chong LY, Head K, Hopkins C, et al. Saline irrigation for chronic rhinosinusitis. Cochrane Database Syst Rev. 2016;4:CD011995. https://doi.org/10.1002/14651858.CD011995.pub2.
9. Wallwork B, Coman W, Mackay-Sim A, et al. A double-blind, randomized, placebo-controlled trial of macrolide in the treatment of chronic rhinosinusitis. Laryngoscope. 2006;116:189–93. https://doi.org/10.1097/01.mlg.0000191560.53555.08.
10. Schembri S, Williamson PA, Short PM, et al. Cardiovascular events after clarithromycin use in lower respiratory tract infections: analysis of two prospective cohort studies. BMJ. 2013;346:f1235. https://doi.org/10.1136/bmj.f1235.
11. Hopkins C, Rimmer J, Lund VJ. Does time to endoscopic sinus surgery impact outcomes in chronic rhinosinusitis? Prospective findings from the National Comparative Audit of Surgery for Nasal Polyposis and Chronic Rhinosinusitis. Rhinology. 2015;53:10–7. https://doi. org/10.4193/Rhin13-217.
12. Hopkins C, Slack R, Lund V, et al. Long-term outcomes from the English national comparative audit of surgery for nasal polyposis and chronic rhinosinusitis. Laryngoscope. 2009;119:2459–65. https://doi.org/10.1002/lary.20653.
13. Hsueh WD, Conley DB, Kim H, et al. Identifying clinical symptoms for improving the symptomatic diagnosis of chronic rhinosinusitis. Int Forum Allergy Rhinol. 2013;3:307–14. https:// doi.org/10.1002/alr.21106.
14. Wu D, Gray ST, Holbrook EH, et al. SNOT-22 score patterns strongly negatively predict chronic rhinosinusitis in patients with headache. Int Forum Allergy Rhinol. 2019;9:9–15. https://doi.org/10.1002/alr.22216.
15. Lal D, Rounds AB, Rank MA, et al. Clinical and 22-item Sino-Nasal Outcome Test symptom patterns in primary headache disorder patients presenting to otolaryngologists with "sinus" headaches, pain or pressure. Int Forum Allergy Rhinol. 2015;5:408–16. https://doi. org/10.1002/alr.21502.
16. Schreiber CP, Hutchinson S, Webster CJ, et al. Prevalence of migraine in patients with a history of self-reported or physician-diagnosed "sinus" headache. Arch Intern Med. 2004;164:1769–72. https://doi.org/10.1001/archinte.164.16.1769.
17. Bellamy JL, Cady RK, Durham PL. Salivary levels of CGRP and VIP in rhinosinusitis and migraine patients. Headache. 2006;46:24–33. https://doi.org/10.1111/j.1526-4610.2006. 00294.x.
18. Eross E, Dodick D, Eross M. The sinus, allergy and migraine study (SAMS). Headache. 2007;47:213–24. https://doi.org/10.1111/j.1526-4610.2006.00688.x.

19. Perry BF, Login IS, Kountakis SE. Nonrhinologic headache in a tertiary rhinology practice. Otolaryngol Head Neck Surg. 2004;130:449–52. https://doi.org/10.1016/j.otohns.2004.01.005.
20. Mehle ME, Kremer PS. Sinus CT scan findings in "sinus headache" migraineurs. Headache. 2008;48:67–71. https://doi.org/10.1111/j.1526-4610.2007.00811.x.
21. Lloyd GA. CT of the paranasal sinuses: study of a control series in relation to endoscopic sinus surgery. J Laryngol Otol. 1990;104:477–81. https://doi.org/10.1017/s0022215100112927.
22. Barham HP, Zhang AS, Christensen JM, et al. Acute radiology rarely confirms sinus disease in suspected recurrent acute rhinosinusitis. Int Forum Allergy Rhinol. 2017;7:726–33. https://doi.org/10.1002/alr.21925.
23. Leung RM, Chandra RK, Kern RC, et al. Primary care and upfront computed tomography scanning in the diagnosis of chronic rhinosinusitis: a cost-based decision analysis. Laryngoscope. 2014;124:12–8. https://doi.org/10.1002/lary.24100.
24. Troeltzsch M, Pache C, Troeltzsch M, et al. Etiology and clinical characteristics of symptomatic unilateral maxillary sinusitis: a review of 174 cases. J Craniomaxillofac Surg. 2015;43:1522–9. https://doi.org/10.1016/j.jcms.2015.07.021.
25. Melen I, Lindahl L, Andreasson L, et al. Chronic maxillary sinusitis. Definition, diagnosis and relation to dental infections and nasal polyposis. Acta Otolaryngol. 1986;101:320–7. https://doi.org/10.3109/00016488609132845.
26. Hoskison E, Daniel M, Rowson JE, et al. Evidence of an increase in the incidence of odontogenic sinusitis over the last decade in the UK. J Laryngol Otol. 2012;126:43–6. https://doi.org/10.1017/S0022215111002568.
27. Lopes LJ, Gamba TO, Bertinato JV, et al. Comparison of panoramic radiography and CBCT to identify maxillary posterior roots invading the maxillary sinus. Dentomaxillofac Radiol. 2016;45:20160043. https://doi.org/10.1259/dmfr.20160043.
28. Maillet M, Bowles WR, McClanahan SL, et al. Cone-beam computed tomography evaluation of maxillary sinusitis. J Endod. 2011;37:753–7. https://doi.org/10.1016/j.joen.2011.02.032.
29. Cartwright S, Hopkins C. Odontogenic Sinusitis an underappreciated diagnosis: Our experience. Clin Otolaryngol. 2016;41:284–5. https://doi.org/10.1111/coa.12499.
30. Shahbazian M, Jacobs R. Diagnostic value of 2D and 3D imaging in odontogenic maxillary sinusitis: a review of literature. J Oral Rehabil. 2012;39:294–300. https://doi.org/10.1111/j.1365-2842.2011.02262.x.
31. Brook I. Sinusitis of odontogenic origin. Otolaryngol Head Neck Surg. 2006;135:349–55. https://doi.org/10.1016/j.otohns.2005.10.059.
32. Mattos JL, Ferguson BJ, Lee S. Predictive factors in patients undergoing endoscopic sinus surgery for odontogenic sinusitis. Int Forum Allergy Rhinol. 2016;6:697–700. https://doi.org/10.1002/alr.21736.
33. Kanagalingam J, Bhatia K, Georgalas C, et al. Maxillary mucosal cyst is not a manifestation of rhinosinusitis: results of a prospective three-dimensional CT study of ophthalmic patients. Laryngoscope. 2009;119:8–12. https://doi.org/10.1002/lary.20037.
34. Ashraf N, Bhattacharyya N. Determination of the "incidental" Lund score for the staging of chronic rhinosinusitis. Otolaryngol Head Neck Surg. 2001;125:483–6. https://doi.org/10.1067/mhn.2001.119324.
35. Cagici CA, Yilmazer C, Hurcan C, et al. Appropriate interslice gap for screening coronal paranasal sinus tomography for mucosal thickening. Eur Arch Otorhinolaryngol. 2009;266:519–25. https://doi.org/10.1007/s00405-008-0786-6.
36. Maska B, Lin GH, Othman A, et al. Dental implants and grafting success remain high despite large variations in maxillary sinus mucosal thickening. Int J Implant Dent. 2017;3:1. https://doi.org/10.1186/s40729-017-0064-8.
37. Jungner M, Legrell PE, Lundgren S. Follow-up study of implants with turned or oxidized surfaces placed after sinus augmentation. Int J Oral Maxillofac Implants. 2014;29:1380–7. https://doi.org/10.11607/jomi.3629.

Correction to: Optimal Pain Management for the Dental Team

Tara Renton

Correction to:
T. Renton (ed.), *Optimal Pain Management for the Dental Team*, BDJ Clinician's Guides,
https://doi.org/10.1007/978-3-030-86634-1

The book was inadvertently published with spelling errors in Figure 1.1 of Chapter 1, Figure 3.1 of Chapter 3, and Table 9.7 of Chapter 9. These errors have been corrected now.

The updated original versions of the chapters can be found at
https://doi.org/10.1007/978-3-030-86634-1_1
https://doi.org/10.1007/978-3-030-86634-1_3
https://doi.org/10.1007/978-3-030-86634-1_9

Printed in the United States
by Baker & Taylor Publisher Services